Health? Your Way !

Dr. Anat Feldman

To my many wonderful clients, who allow me to be part of their personal miraculous journey. Thank you for inspiring me to learn and grow, both professionally and personally. To my precious family, who with love and patience, acceptance and tenderness, enabled all this to emerge.

Table of Contents

Chapter II: Nutrition, Awareness and Body-Image. Primary thoughts and some proven facts: Eating smart for your health (128)

Chapter III: The power of the Mind, Therapy and Change. Primary thought: The power of your mind over your body (202)

"Man is condemned to be free; because once thrown into the world, he is responsible for everything he does".
Jean-Paul Sartre.

Before you begin

Humankind is on a quest for a longer, healthier, and better life. It's an issue well discussed on TV shows, magazines, books, and websites. It seems as if every second a new health study appears before the public to bring THE answer for our perplexity about what is good for us. We are not necessarily here to find the "best answer for you". This would be too presumptuous, since no one can really give the "best answer for you"... but you. I do base this book on the strong supposition that the right path for health, happiness, and abundance is so personal that only the individual himself is responsible for finding and embracing the "best answer". I wish to inspire you to seek health and happiness the way that best suits you, while taking into consideration "all areas of life" and the strong rapport between three components that determine our health: Fitness - "work-out", Nutrition -"eating smart" and Mind -"work-in" mentally, emotionally, and spiritually. This is what Gymind is all about, a holistic way of life, a methodology of Doing and Being, of Physiology and Philosophy, my "raison d'être" as a trainer and a therapist for the past decade.

Knowledge means power; information provides the tools, means, and understanding. So while research and recent fitness-nutrition-mind studies do form the groundwork of this book, they are not alone. Personal stories of wonderful individuals who are in that constant search for health consistently emerge throughout this book. We may recognize ourselves between the lines, we may strongly identify with some, perhaps related to their situation – only to be inspired to take charge over our life and take action. We must take the time to know ourselves, listen to our body, our needs, our soul, and act upon this knowledge to find the right path for us. Muriel, Aida, Oliver, Maya, Irene, Barak, Belle, Leroy, Tamara, Matt, Bethany, Hanna, Ili, Emma, Tami, Liana and Ave embrace Gymind as a way of life. Those individuals, diverse in age, gender, and goals in life, whose stories are shaded in grey along with other tips and guidelines, are for now anonymous to us. At the end of this book we will know them a little better, but more importantly, we will, hopefully, know ourselves better.

This book consists of three chapters: 1. Fitness, 2. Nutrition 3. Mind, apparently separated, yet strongly connected. Not only by the personal stories that trace those individual's path of health, but also by the belief that fitness-nutrition-mind are by definition and undeniably related, to the extent that HEALTH as we seek and strive for is incomplete without any one of them.

Fitness wise: What is the best work-out plan for good health? Is there a special fitness program for men, women, and children or is there a "master plan" adequate for all? Can one become an "athlete" or embrace the joy of exercising and sports activity at an advanced age? Is it ever "too late" to begin? Can "bad habits" be changed? How can one get rid of "limiting beliefs" such as: "I will always be fat"; "Nothing ever works out for me"; "I hate to work out"?

Nutrition-wise: What is "eating smart" all about? How can one make the right choices with all the "forbidden temptations" out there? Is there a special nutrition program for men, women, and children, or is there a "master plan" adequate for all? Is the combination of working-out and eating-smart enough to lose weight and keep it off? What role does "self-image" play in the process of losing weight and maintaining a healthy life-style? How can we use visualization and imagination in order to improve physical performance, upgrade our eating habits, or even manifest abundance?

Mind-wise: How strong are "external affirmations" (repetition of words and phrases, such as "I am healthy, I am strong, etc.") in order to achieve abundance and good health? What part does the subconscious mind play in the process of attaining our goals in life? How can one "work-in" in order to hold on to those goals and accomplish more to come? How can one avoid "toxic emotions" and clear our soul of negative feelings in order to heal physically and maintain good health?

The first chapter: "Fitness, work-outs, know your body" opens with the fundamental understanding, so important for further discussions, that body-soul-mind-spirit are inseparable. When we honor our body as a whole, listen to its needs, physically and mentally, we are in better communication with ourselves; hence we get to know ourselves better, then accept and love our body as a whole. This is the key for success, for a better life, for health. Only then we can dive into a profound discussion about the physiology of exercise and the importance of movement, of walking or running; BMI as an indicator for illness; recommended fitness plans according to your age and according to your goal. This chapter may serve as a manual of exercises encouraging us to take care and take charge over our body: "20 minutes and you're done" fitness programs to work all muscle groups and serve as an adequate work-out plan in the busy life we manage. In an era of sedentary life-style, an important place is reserved for children's activity and the importance of proper physical education at a young age, starting at home and at school; this chapter does not exclude the importance of breathing and relaxation for balance and mental well-being. It mainly encourages us to know our body, set a physical goal, and choose the suitable fitness plan for our needs.

The second chapter, "Nutrition, Awareness, and Body-Image", sheds some light on the importance of eating smart, based on the belief that the better the fuel, the better our body runs. It seeks to inspire us with some nutrition plans according to our goals, whether it's to lose weight, gain more muscle, or maintain healthy eating habits. This chapter raises one of the most important notions according to the Gymind path, that of Awareness, that along with Responsibility and Choice, helps us with a better understanding of our body, our nutritional needs at any age, and even provides us with some exciting tools of how to "change the automaton" and take control over our nutritional choices. An important place is kept for children's nutrition in this disturbing era of children's obesity, along with the critical need to maintain, or create if necessary, a healthy body-image. It's in this chapter that we will learn more about the creation of Gymind as a methodology, through personal experiences. This chapter calls us once again to know ourselves and to choose a nutrition plan that fits our needs.

The third chapter, "The power of the mind, therapy and change" develops almost naturally out of the two other chapters. Where we earlier only fleetingly touched upon the endless possibilities of our mind as far as changing the automaton, embracing new habits, using mind techniques at the gym or empowering ourselves with an improved self-image, this profound. magical, exciting chapter goes even further to explore the power that our mind possesses over our body. With the premise that "anything is possible", we are hereby invited to stop insisting on our limitations, "be at cause" and be responsible in our mind for that change we wish and strive for. We will learn what NLP is all about and encounter some tools to reprogram our thoughts; we will learn how to better communicate with ourselves and with others; we will learn that "it's never too late to have a happy childhood" thanks to Time Line Therapy. With EFT we will learn to release the toxic and negative emotions that don't serve us any longer, and never really did. We will not exclude the spiritual yet so important part of this book, suitable for children and adults, the spiritual side of our Being, through meditations and the "sixth sense" for holistic health. We will climb all the way up to the "seventh plane of existence" to find inner peace and healing using Theta waves of the brain. As in the two previous chapters, this chapter will also call upon us to know ourselves, take charge and set a goal to manifest health and abundance, thanks to those magnificent tools.

Chapter I

Fitness, work-out, know your body

Primary thoughts: Body and soul, the same entity
We must agree, along with modern medicine as well as ancient
spiritual Zen and Buddhism, on this indisputable argument in order
to establish a thesis: Body-soul-mind-spirit are strongly connected,
inseparable, so influenced by one another, up to a point where we
can refer to them as one: The SELF. You will easily relate to this
theory. Take, for instance, a non-ulcer stomach ache one suffers
from. According to the Mayo Clinic approach (2011), conventional
medicine knows to ask nowadays: Have you felt stressed lately? What
do you "keep inside"? What is the "mental source" of this pain? And
then, how changes in diet and lifestyle as well as exercise, cognitive-
behavioral therapy and mindfulness-based stress reduction can help
your doctor find the adequate cure and sometimes avoid unnecessary
medical interventions. (Larzelere, 2008). No need to go that far,
though. Hunched shoulders and a wrong posture can indicate weak
back extensors. It can also be as a result, or the exterior reflection, of
low self-esteem, shyness, or mental trauma of any sort. Shahidi (2013)
found that upper trapezius muscles are selectively activated by
psychosocial stress independent of changes in concentration or
posture. Treatment can be dual: Exercising and toning up the
Latissimus Dorsi may strengthen the spirit. It's also the mental
therapy that aims to lift the spirit that will bring higher self-esteem,
making one stand straight and improve posture. Examples of that
sort are countless. We encounter them frequently; we have all
experienced the strong connection between body and soul.

Carved into the pillars of the Temple of Apollo at Delphi were two
famous phrases: γνῶθι σεαυτόν (gnōthi seautón = "Know thyself")
and μηδέν ἄγαν (mēdén ágan = "Nothing in excess"). Knowledge is

Power. And understanding is the key, not only for attaining good health but also for keeping up the results for many years to come.

Define YOUR health. We may have lost our inner compass; hence the goal is to find a more accurate compass to guide us on the path for good health. According to Agus (2012), we will not be able to enjoy the benefits of what he refers to as "personalized medicine" until we get up close and personal with ourselves. Nothing about health is "one-size-fits-all" so until we know how to do our own "fitting", we won't be able to live the long and happy life that's awaiting us.

"People say that…", "I heard at the gym that…" "I read this article where they said that…" "Everybody knows this is good for you…" Phrases we hear and may use all the time in order to make a point, phrases I strongly resent:
Nancy, a former client, with a high awareness of health and good nutrition, (who needed my support to maintain that healthy life-style), identified herself as "somewhat allergic to soy products". She couldn't quite put a finger of what exactly but it seemed that each time she ate a product which contained soy, she felt bloated and heavy, so she tried to avoid them. When she moved to a different city, I referred her to another nutritionist-herbalist. After her first session with him she called me complaining that he had prescribed some soy products in her diet. I wrote him a polite email underlining the fact he had already known: Nancy cannot bear soy products. His response was shocking to me: "A billion Chinese who eat soy products can't be mistaken".

Miller, 32, married and a father of 2, expressed his wish to start running long distances. "What kind of activity are you currently into?" I asked. "Swimming "he answered. "I swim three to four times a week for a distance of 4-5 km". "What do you need to run for?" I asked at once. "People say running is the best…"

We did put Miller on an adequate running program, but he never forgot his real passion and despite his primary wish to replace swimming with running, he continues to swim twice a week.

We should define our personal health, physically, emotionally, spiritually, mentally. It's only in the third chapter that we deal with the study of the Mind, for it's essential to begin with the "physical", our body, the closest "thing" we possess, that "tool" that holds, guards, and interacts with the mind. Our soul and mind are "located" inside our body. We also agree that a dialogue between mind and body exists. Certainly, it may be easier to cure a visible bruise than to mend a broken heart or cure a phobia of any sort. However, during the course of handling the "physical", we can more easily delve into the "mental". Many of my clients began their health process with the "Gym" part and only later integrated the "Mind" part. That may be the reason why this book begins with the physiology of the human body, the "work-out", and not necessarily the "work-in".

Work-out for good health; reduce sedentary behavior

The human body is "born" to move. The first steps we take, jumping around as kids, jogging, dancing to music, even swimming, are all actions that come very naturally to us. Kids typically perform squats and deadlifts without anyone having to show them how. When a tot picks up the ball, he squats down from his hips with his chest up high and lifts it without the slightest bend in his back or any overt awareness of the movement pattern. It happens very naturally, so that he does not even have any idea what he has done (Kavalo, 2011). It is only during the past few decades that it has become possible for people to go through life with minimal physical activity. The modern way of living promotes comfort and well-being in a less energy-demanding environment (Chaput, 2011). So most people nowadays don't use their bodies to their full capabilities (Agin, 2008). Sitting down most of the day, despite a strenuous morning workout, can be as bad as or worse than smoking, states Agus (2012). McGinnis, (1993) adds to that, asserting that the most important modifiable determinants of cancer risk, (besides use of tobacco), are weight control, dietary choices, and levels of physical activity. One-third of the more than 572,000 cancer deaths that occur in the United States each year can be attributed to diet and physical activity habits (Lawrence, 2012). An important study conducted by CPS-II, the Cancer Prevention Study II (Alpa V. Patel, 2012), shows the surprising damages of sitting. This study, which began in 1982, found that sitting for six or more hours daily can elevate chances of dying from cancer and other major diseases, even if one maintains a healthy weight, and even if you are a non-smoker. "Just sitting for 2.5 hours less each day would result in an extra energy expenditure of 350 kcal per day", Ravussin (2005) calculates, which could translate into preventing the gain of extra kilograms. With the right practice, "natural movements" we have lost over the years usually return, and with them come increased strength, flexibility, and, of course, functionality (Kavalo, 2011).

Almost any activity can count as exercise. From walking and dancing to swimming or biking. Staying fit means listening to our body and learning to what makes us feel the best. It is important to be patient if we take on strenuous aerobic activity or strength training. Trying to up the intensity too quickly can lead to injury and loss of motivation.

"Knowing is not enough; we must apply. Willing is not enough; we must do." (Johann Wolfgang von Goethe)

We know exercise is a Must. We wish to embrace an active life-style, and our mind is set in the right direction. Our body needs to move, our muscles need to work hard, to the point of fatigue in order to rebuild themselves and grow stronger. Our body craves "to do"; it craves pain, movement, and resistance (Agin, 2008). A study from the University's Department of Physical Therapy (Marcus, 2008), shows how patients with diabetes who participate in a program combining aerobic and high-force eccentric resistance exercise demonstrate improvements in glucose control, physical performance, and body fat composition. The influence of physical activity on brain plasticity might have consequences not only for memory and other cognitive functions, but also has implications for many different psychiatric and neurologic conditions through a set of common biological pathways (Kirk, 2013).

Hanna, 22, came to my studio four years ago. Her goal was to lose some weight and to be in shape. She "hated" sports (so she claimed), needed a personal trainer to get her motivated, and "dragged" herself 40 kilometers to meet me once a week for an hour of Gymind session. In her mind she knew she had "to DO" but basically she needed a constant push. For months and months that was the case: An hour of training session once a week, combined with healthy nutrition that she maintained during the day. Things have changed during that time. Hanna slowly "absorbed" the importance of "DOING". I am not sure if she "fell in love" with fitness activities (we are still talking about it), but she certainly slowly embraced the joy of "feeling" her muscles, appreciating physical resistance and pain. She aims for a work-out 6 days a week, (on her own, at home), for exactly 20 minutes, not longer and enjoys the optimum doze of exercise her body needs for maintaining balanced weight and good health.

DOING is so important that even minor changes will suffice. The Cancer Prevention Study II suggests we get a daily dose of movement:

Set an alarm on your computer to remind you to stand up for a few minutes once every hour for better blood flow.

Work standing up, just like Thomas Jefferson and Ernest Hemingway, among others who used a raised desk so they could stand while working.

Skip interoffice phone and email, so when you want to discuss something with a colleague at work you are compelled to get up and walk to their desk instead.

Use your feet instead of sitting in a car when you need to run an errand within walking distance.

Choose leisure activities that don't involve sitting, such as dancing, bowling, or museums, instead of movie theatres, concerts or attending a sports event as a spectator.

Body Mass Index (BMI): A reliable index for health?

The school nurse called me a year ago just after a routine physical check-up that my youngest son (a very athletic and active 7-year-old) underwent with his class mates. "Dr. Feldman, your son is over-weight; you should take him to see his doctor and a nutritionist". "Have you seen my son?" I asked in a pleasant tone. "I do not remember specifically", she answered. " I simply read from a chart, I have his BMI results in front of me".

BMI is an approximate measure of body fat based on height and weight. First proposed by the Belgian statistician Adolphe Quételet in 1835, it is calculated by the formula: Weight /(height)^2, kg/m^2. Its popularity derives from its simplicity and the fact that weight and height are easily measured. Standard categories of BMI: 18.5-<25 (normal weight), 25-<30 (overweight), and >=30 (obese) (Kabat, 2012). A recent study, based on another study conducted in 2005 by the same researchers (Flegal, 2013), further subdivided the last category into 30-<35 (class 1), 35-<40 (class 2), and >=40 (class 3) and found that compared to normal weight individuals, those in the overweight category had a lower risk of dying of any cause, and those in the obese category had an elevated risk. No grand news there. However, more than half of those in the obese category were in class 1, and these individuals had no increased risk of dying compared to normal weight individuals. Class 2 and 3 individuals did have a significantly elevated risk of death. Kabat concluded (2013) that being overweight actually appeared beneficial and that the ill effects of obesity were limited to the very obese. Back in 2005, researchers also studied the effect of exercise and active life style. In 2005, when it was first published that being overweight was associated with lower mortality, researchers got tremendous amount of negative feedback. Since that study, dozens of others have reached the same conclusion, even if it was hard for researchers and the public to accept.

It seems as if BMI does not tell us all we need to know. This is because BMI does not distinguish between fat mass and lean mass (muscle, water, bone, internal organs). Someone who is physically fit can have a higher BMI due to having greater than average muscle mass. My son's BMI indicates nothing but his body mass, and nothing about his muscle tone or fat percentage.

A predictor of illness

Many doctors and nutritionists do use BMI as an index for good health, but how is it really useful in predicting long-term good health?

BMI, while not a perfect indicator, does correlate moderately well with body fat. So the fact that BMI has increased over the past decades in the U.S is telling us something, adds Kabat, (2013). Even more significant is the fact that the proportion of the population in the very obese category has increased. Moreover, the increasing prevalence of high BMI in childhood is a worrying phenomenon (Flegal, 2013). In spite of its limitations, BMI is a strong predictor of a person's risk of diabetes. According to the Centers for Disease Control and Prevention (CDC, 2013), between 1995 and 2010 the age-adjusted prevalence of diabetes in U.S. adults increased from 4.4% to 8.2%, and its prevalence is projected to continue to increase in the future.

"Picture" your weight: "Happy Feet"

Going through a process of acquiring a healthy life-style is easier with a supportive friend. According to Huberty (2013), and research she conducted at the University of Nebraska-Omaha, (polling more than 300 women who'd been exercising regularly for longer than a year), recruiting a friend to join in your quest for a healthy and active life-style makes that process more appealing.

The HAPPY FEET method was born out of those needs. When clients needed the extra-support from their trainer outside the walls of the studio and during their everyday life.

When do you use HAPPY FEET?

When you are unable to attend a Gymind session or use the scale at the studio.

When you attend a Gymind evening session and consequently get an "incorrect" weight, a "false" result after a long day of eating and drinking. Recommendations are for a once-a-week morning weigh-in. (Hart, 2013).

In between Gymind sessions, three days after a weigh-in, when you want to get a glimpse of your progress and receive an "extra-push".

HAPPY FEET are pictures sent as MMS, (picture messages), via What'sApp or email, in different colors shapes, and sizes (as shown in the picture). They "cuddle" the number they hold, act proud and excited about the results, sometimes promise: "Next time will be better", sometimes cheer you up: "The effort has paid off!". They are "happy feet" who carry our physical and mental weight and burden. They deserve to be heard, they deserve to be treated well. We don't only listen to them, get connected with their needs creating a Body-Mind-Head-to-Toe connection, being our own best friends, but we also get to share that interaction with a friend and get extra support.

Behind every picture there is a man or a woman engaged in the process of health; to that connection between the SELF and the weight, to the connection between what might be a reflection of that "bingeing" the previous weekend and the gain of a half of a kilo as a result. Those Happy Feet take responsibility; they face reality, fully aware and exposed.

Jasmine, a 15-year-old girl, came to see me at her regular scheduled time: Tuesday at 16:00 pm. She had been expecting to see a major weight loss after a week of balanced nutrition. The result was disappointing. "It may be your muscle mass", I suggested comfortingly (since we had been engaged in core training), "or it may be the amount of water you drank just before our session". "Did you eat salty foods yesterday?". "You know there is a difference between a morning weigh-in and an evening weigh-in. What did YOUR scale show this morning?"

The next morning Jasmine sent me a picture of her HAPPY FEET holding the low number she had hoped to see.

Remember that each scale is calibrated differently so we should always compare results from the same scale.

How does it work?
We weigh in once a week, in the morning. I recommend a Monday-morning-weigh-in to control the potential week-end's over eating. Use the same clothes every time or just weigh in fully naked (the picture does not show that). Click the camera and send your Happy Feet picture to someone who is prepared to cheer you up if needed. You can simply keep that picture on your desk top or your smartphone.

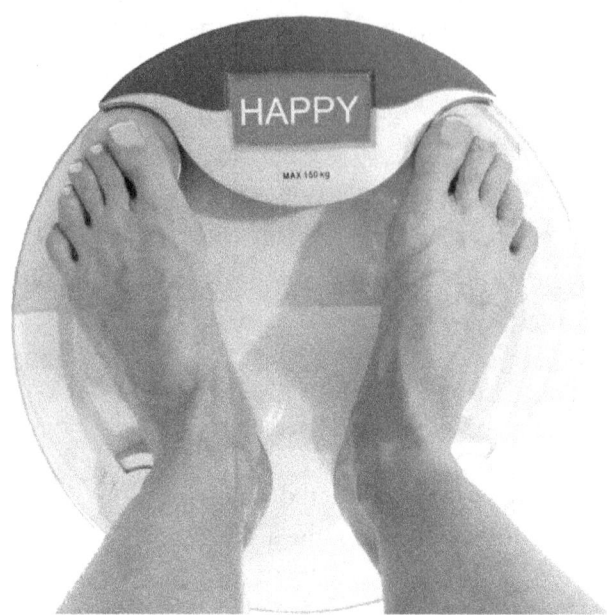

"Happy feet"

Flexible Mind and the challenge to run

Success in weight loss begins in the mind, when we make a conscious decision to change behaviors. The term "flexible mind" can relate to memory strategies or emotional stability (Colzato, 2006, 2010). In this book we refer to it not necessarily in that sense. The term "flexible mind" is defined here as a cognitive flexibility, a switch in thinking, whether that is specifically based on a switch in rules or broadly based on a need to switch one's previous beliefs or thoughts to new situations (Scott, 1962). When a person is "chained" to old habits, beliefs, conceptions about himself and his life, but he is open to "recruiting" his mind to create a change, (because he wants the change, no matter how extreme and distant it may be from what he knows and is familiar with), he uses the flexibility of his mind.

Meet Aida, her broken thigh (and spirit)

Aida, 45, married, and a mom of three, came to my studio three years ago. Her daughter had been seeing me for over a year prior to our encounter for weight-loss and nutrition consult. Aida had always wanted to make a change in her life just like her daughter did. She was finally ready and determined to make a change.

First encounter: 29.11.2011

Physical parameters: 1.65, 72.7 kg.

Aida's goals: Losing weight; being in shape; embracing a healthy life-style; running.

Aida's first wish, expressed with shining eyes (even before she sat down on the couch in our first encounter) was: "I wish I could run". It was then and there that I firmly told her: "Great, let's step out of the studio and go take your first run". The switch was made instantly. And over the next four weeks, with the proper physical practice, a solid training program, and mostly with the proper state of mind- a runner was born.

Aida's fear of running was justified. She was not much of a sporty person as a child, but it was a traumatic event at the age of 19 that led her to a complete loss of trust in her body, so that the ability of her legs to carry her ("running her") was questionable. When Aida was 19 years old, she had experienced abnormal pains in her thighs. For months doctors could not find the root cause of the pain, until a random US showed a tumor in her mid-thigh. Aida was operated and the tumor was taken out. But the worst was still ahead. One day, while standing on one leg, Aida heard a loud "crack", fell down, and found herself with a broken thigh. "An unfortunate rare condition" as the doctors stated, which compelled her to undergo long, excruciating operations. Aida lost not only her freedom during those long months of recuperating, but at the age of 19 she lost her confidence. "I did not trust my left thigh" she said. "At the age of 19 I was trapped in an old treacherous-back-stabber of a body".

From a couch potato to an athlete: Can you become a sports lover?

Notice how people tend to carry signs that (they assume) define them. "I hate sports", "I am not made for jogging" or "I would never neglect my sedentary behavior no matter how hard I try to", would be a small sample of how the signs that people had created at some point in their life and still insist on carrying, control their life and give a distorted definition of who they "really" are. Those signs suit them. They have what Stevenson (2008) calls a "secondary gain". Those people "earn" something: permission to rest, maybe some sympathy from society and surely some attention. Those signs create a form of identity, a definition of the self, which even if false or negative, still makes them feel at ease with the comforting knowledge of who they are. Their subconscious mind has created at some point that "decision": "I am a couch potato", and there you have it. A person who is out of shape, flabby, doesn't feel so great, and it is harder and harder for him to move around and do the basic things, becomes a typical "couch potato". The good news is: He can become a "former couch potato" and even a real athlete.

The first step would be finding that WILL for a change. Just like Aida who was determined about her will to run, something she had only dreamed about for years after her injury; just like Oliver the 12-year-old we will encounter later on in this chapter who said repeatedly "I need a change".

The second step would be to acknowledge that a change CAN be made. Communicating with the subconscious mind will be discussed in-depth in Chapter 3, but acknowledging the fact that the person who created those signs can easily put them away would sometimes be enough to achieve a complete change.

And then, by DOING long enough - a new and improved habit will emerge.

How to change habits?

The dictionary definition of habit is "an acquired pattern of behavior that often occurs automatically". Our habits, mostly automatic and natural, shape many of our actions in life. If a person were to ask himself: "Why do I come home from work and sit in front of the TV instead of going for a walk?", the answer would be "Because I'm used to doing it" and it would also be a habit. Our brain works by generating electrochemical impulses. Different nerve cells and parts of our brain communicate with one another through impulses. Every time we do something new, our brain generates a sequence of impulses, which travel through our nerve cells. The nerve cells through which those impulses travel are called a neural pathway. With each new task, the brain creates a new neural pathway, and every time we perform that same action in that same way, our brain will use this same neural pathway. This is called "brain plasticity" and refers to the ability to reorganize itself to adapt to changes in the functional system. The more we perform the same exact action, the more comfortable our brain will be using that neural pathway, which means it becomes a comfortable habit for us. (Frackowiak, 1997). A study from Brown Medical School in Rhode Island found, after a close study from 1995 to 2003, that the eating and exercise habits of successful weight losers do change for the better. The variables associated with long-term maintenance of weight loss were the same: Continued consumption of a low-calorie diet with moderate fat intake, limited consumption of fast food, and high levels of physical activity (Phelan, 2006).

So we can use the power of habit to eradicate bad choices and create good ones.

Identify your current established habits in relation to health, fitness, and nutrition. This will clarify which ones need improvement.

Understand the power you have to change things. That same force that has kept you stuck is the same force that will help you succeed.

Design the new habit to replace the old one. We can't eliminate the old habit without putting something in its place. In doing so, we are left with a void, and the brain will revert to the old habit to fill that void.

Consciously create the new habit in a way that will be easy to implement. For Aida, running nearby her house every evening was a convenient enough new habit she was happy to adopt.

Begin now. Not tomorrow. And keep up the new pattern until it becomes a habit, for at least 21 consecutive days. Why 21 days? It may well come from a book published in 1960 by a plastic surgeon. Dr. Maxwell Maltz noticed that amputees took on average 21 days to adjust to the loss of a limb, and he argued that people take 21 days to adjust to any major life changes. Studies, however, show that it takes 66 days for a neural pathway to solidify in your mind. (Lally, 2010). The new habit may feel awkward at the beginning but this will subside as the new habit becomes more comfortable.

Think about what you actually can do. Walking, for example. Walking to the next room. Embark on a walking program. If you are physically unable to walk 30 minutes, walk 15 minutes. Even if you do just 5 minutes a day, start.

The Swish Pattern

The swish pattern is a very simple and effective way to create an objective and favorable image of yourself that produces immediate results in specific troublesome situations. In this case, changing a bad habit by using the ability of the mind to adapt to a new behavior you create. Swish patterns are for the purpose of creating momentum toward a compelling future, hence, install choices for a new way of life.

Get the picture that represents the habit or the situation you would like to change. When you think of that bad habit, do you have a picture?

Get the picture of the type of person you would like to be. How would you like to be instead? When you think of that, do you have a picture?

Change the visual intensity of the desired state and make the picture brighter, bigger, and closer. Do whatever you need to create it better for you, for the most "real" or most positive Kinesthetic. For example: See yourself in control over your body, in charge, feeling happy and content.

Bring back the old picture.

Insert in the lower left-hand corner a small dark picture of the desired state.

Simultaneously have the picture of the current state rapidly shrink and recede to a distant point while the dark picture is blown up into a full screen. This can be accompanied by a SWISH sound

Repeat for five times and make sure you have a break between each Swish Pattern so as not to loop them. (Clear the screen or open and then close your eyes). (Stevenson, 2007).

It only took Aida the fraction of a minute to digest my suggestion, make a switch, and go out for a run. It took her a few weeks and a whole training session to maintain a 3 km. smooth run, but her mind was ready, it was already "there", in action. By the end of week 4, Aida was ready for a smooth 20 minute run.

Aida's training program

Week 1, Week 2, Week 3, Week 4.

Sun.	Mon.	Tue.	Wed.	Thurs.	Fri.	Sat.
2 min. walk	2 min. walk	rest	1 min. walk	rest	1 min. walk	rest
30 sec. light jogging	30 sec. light jogging		1 min. light jogging		1.30 min. light jogging	
2 min. fast walk	2 min. fast walk		2 min. fast walk		2 min. fast walk	
30 sec. light jogging	30 sec. light jogging		1 min. light jogging		1 min. light jogging	
2 min. fast walk	2 min. fast walk		2 min. walking		2 min. walking	
30 sec. light jogging	30 sec. light jogging		1 min. light jogging		1 min. light jogging	
2 min. walking and end of training	2 min. walking and end of training		2 min. walking and end of training		2 min. walking and end of training	
9.30 min.	9.30 min.		10 min.		10.30 min.	

Sun.	Mon.	Tue.	Wed.	Thurs.	Fri.	Sat.
2 min. walk	2 min. walk	rest	2 min. walk	rest	2 min. walk	rest
1.30 min. light jogging	1.30 min. light jogging		2 min. light jogging		2 min. light jogging	
1 min. fast walk	1 min. fast walk		1 min. fast walk		2 min. fast walk	
1.30 min. light jogging	1.30 min. light jogging		2 min. light jogging		2 min. light jogging	
1 min. fast walk	1 min. fast walk		1 min. walking		1 min. walking	
1.30 min. light jogging	1.30 min. light jogging		2 min. light jogging		2 min. light jogging	
2 min. walking and end of training	2 min. walking and end of training		2 min. walking and end of training		2 min. walking and end of training	
10.30 min.	10.30 min.		12 min.		13 min.	

Sun.	Mon.	Tue.	Wed.	Thurs.	Fri.	Sat.
2 min. walk	2 min. walk	rest	2 min. walk	rest	2 min. walk	rest
3 min. light jogging	3 min. light jogging		3 min. light jogging		4 min. light jogging	
1 min. fast walk	1 min. fast walk		1 min. fast walk		1 min. fast walk	
3 min. light jogging	3 min. light jogging		3 min. light jogging		4 min. light jogging	
1 min. walking	1 min. walking		1 min. walking		1 min. walking	
3 min. light jogging	3 min. light jogging		3 min. light jogging		4 min. light jogging	
2 min. walking and end of training	2 min. walking and end of training		2 min. walking and end of training		2 min. walking and end of training	
15 min.	15 min.		15 min.		18 min.	

Sun.	Mon.	Tue.	Wed.	Thurs.	Fri.	Sat.
2 min. walk	2 min. walk	rest	2 min. walk	rest	2 min. walk	rest
4 min. light jogging	4 min. light jogging		5 min. light jogging		8 min. light jogging	
1 min. fast walk	1 min. fast walk		1 min. fast walk		1 min. fast walk	
4 min. light jogging	4 min. light jogging		5 min. light jogging		8 min. light jogging	
1 min. walking	1 min. walking		1 min. walking		1 min. fast walking	
4 min. light jogging	4 min. light jogging		5 min. light jogging		2 min. walking and end of training	
2 min. walking and end of training	2 min. walking and end of training		2 min. walking and end of training			
18 min.	18 min.		21 min.		22 min.	

A training session to support your run

"Pain is inevitable, suffering is optional" wrote Haruki Murrakami, (2005), in his fascinating "What I Talk about when I Talk about Running." It's well known that in order to improve running abilities as far as cardio-vascular capacities and mental skills, we need to practice and engage in…running. Even 30 minutes twice a week at an average ratio improves physiological parameters and helps maintain good health. This training program complements your regular run and helps you improve your capacities, embrace pain and avoid suffering.

Several highlights:

Maintain balanced and smart nutrition.

Don't give up on stretching, especially after you complete your work-out.

Make sure you also work on your abdominal muscles, back and upper body. They all take part in running, and strengthening them is good for your balance and posture during your run and long after.

Practice both aerobic training and anaerobic training, (each one of them twice a week), to improve your run and perfect it.

Visualize this: While you jog, think about a circle or a ball that rolls. Try to avoid a "vertical" running which makes your ankle "fastened" on the ground and your whole run look like a square trying to roll. So keep your abs tucked-in and let your body lean a bit forward. That's the way to save energy while letting gravity take effect. Relax your arms, yet keep them at a 90 degree angle. Swing them by your sides instead of swinging them across your body, which makes the torso twist.

Exercise no. 1: Strong knee lifts

Starting position: Place your left foot on the step. The right ankle holds a 2 kg weight.

Lift your right knee towards the chest and go back to starting position. Make sure your abs are tight and remember to breathe throughout the exercise.

How many? 10 consecutive lifts of the right knee, 10 left, twice in a row.

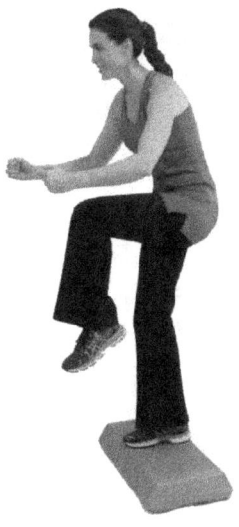

Exercise no 2: Power Jumps

Starting position: Stand on both sides of the step, knees slightly bent. Place weight on both feet.

Perform a "soft" jump with both feet on the step, place right foot in front of the left on landing. Get off of the step back to starting position, (without jumping).

How many? Change position of feet on the step, 14 times in a row.

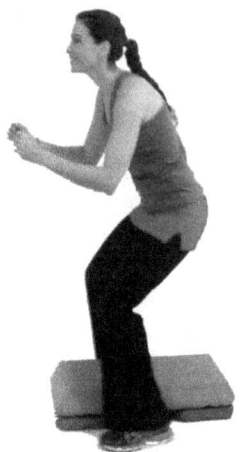

Exercise no. 3: Lunge back

Starting position: Start by standing on the step, spreading your feet slightly apart. Place weight on both feet.

Take one step back with your right leg and place foot pad on the ground. Maintain your balance. Stay in position for two seconds and get back on the step to starting position.

How many? Twice with right foot, twice with left, 3 times in a row.

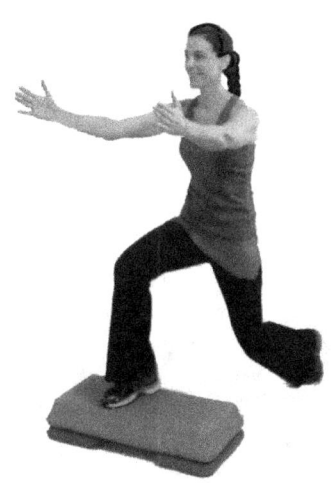

Exercise no. 4: Focus on your thigh

Starting position: Sit on the step; place your palms on the step for support, as they are turned towards your body. Place your feet on the ground, bend your knees.

Lift your right knee towards your chest then straighten it forward so that both knees are aligned. Make sure you flex your foot. Go back to starting position.

How many? 10 with right leg, 10 with left, twice in a row.

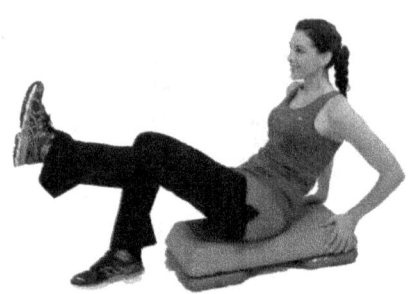

Walking or running?

Thousands of doctors recommend walking. Hundreds of studies extol its benefits. It's simple, enjoyable, and can be done virtually anywhere. When it's properly done, walking can blast away fat as fast as jogging, maybe faster. Even better, speed walking is easier on our joints, since we hit the ground with less than half the force we do when we jog. As a result, we are less likely to have our fitness goals sidelined by soreness or injury (Yeager, 2011). For those who walk yet have pangs for conscience for not being a jogger, a group of researchers from Mississippi University, (Loftin, 2008) has determined that walking and running are the same as far as calorie expenditure, as long as the distance is fixed. Early results from a 2006 study found that walking, (not abdominal exercise specifically), reduced the size of subcutaneous abdominal fat cells, (cell size predicts type 2 diabetes), according to a leading author. Moderate exercise reduced cell size by about 18% in 45 obese women over a 20-week period. Diet alone did not appear to affect cell size. So what is better? Is walking "enough" to maintain a healthy life-style and enjoy a healthy body? Or just like in Aida's case, there is "nothing that compares to jogging" in order to make us feel that "rush" in our body?

A journey of a thousand miles begins with a single step (Lao-Tzu)

"Walking is man's best medicine" said Hippocrates, the father of modern medicine, and boy, was he right! Walking burns calories; eases back pain; slims waist; lowers blood pressure; reduces levels of bad cholesterol; reduces heart attack risks; enhances stamina and energy; lessens anxiety and tension. Hormones called endorphins serve as natural pain killers and they have positive a psychological effect, producing a boost that lasts for hours after a good walk. Walking improves muscle tone and slows down osteoporosis bone loss. Walking can be done everywhere, at any given time and on a daily basis, according to Sportline's Guide to Walking, 2007. Finishing a walk on a day when we had to drag ourselves out the door gives us a sense of victory. A walk of 20 minutes is enough to improve the way we feel about ourselves, and it gives us a sense of achievement. We are "born to walk". It's easy to do, healthy, available and free (Galloway, 2006). When choosing walking over running as an activity, we even avoid this "Pain" that Murrakami, (2005), talks about. It's all about pure joy, simplicity, and flow.

When we cover a certain distance on foot, we receive a unique sense of satisfaction which brings us back to our roots. Primitive human ancestors defined and nurtured uniquely human traits during constant migrations. Our intuition or gut instinct is engaged when we shift into the brain's right hemisphere. As we walk at a pace within our capabilities, we return to some "primitive" areas in the brain which have subconscious judgment capabilities and other powers we don't usually use. So miles into the walk we take a certain problem, and we think of it with a mix of images, laughs, inner thoughts, so that the right brain ends up by entertaining us (Galloway, 2006).

Walking in the morning may give a boost of energy to begin our day with, to both our mind and body. Taking a walk during lunch time makes one more productive and capable of facing the rest of the day. At evening time, especially three hours before bedtime, walking can improve the quality of sleep. It also helps speed up metabolism. Sure, says Fenton, (2006), "formal" exercise such as going to the gym or taking a fitness class is great. But what we do in everyday life matters tremendously.

Pedometer to count your steps

We must trust walking; BELIEVE that walking can make the difference in our life – and it will. It will provide self-confidence, balance and even emotional calm in life. Eat smart every day and trust walking, and for the health of it - build a daily habit. (Fenton, 2001). The Gymind method is all about making it as comfortable as we can. It's all about availability and the way we integrate movement and physical activity in our everyday life. A small and affordable device can help us do just that.

In our busy lifestyle, people complain they don't have the time or energy to take a walk every day. That's why keeping a Pedometer is so recommended. It's not a matter of speed, power or how long you take the walk; it's only a matter of counting the steps we make per day. 10,000 of them is the number to reach. A 15-week program research (Morgan, 2010) shows that taking 10,000 steps per day improves cardiovascular performances and positively influences many variables that are indicators of health, fitness and psychological well-being.

An innovative online pedometer program was developed by Dr. James Hill at the Center for Human Nutrition at the University of Colorado Health Science Center in Denver. The goal is for participants to increase their activity by 2000 steps per day and to decrease consumption by 100 calories per day, in order to prevent "creeping obesity".

Ravussin notes (2005), that American adults gain an average of 1.8 pounds per year, "the whole idea is, if we can get people more active, we can greatly improve health and reduce weight gain". America as a nation is recruited to control this burning issue by motivating the American people to walk in www.americaonthemove.com.[1] Using a pedometer it's simple to track, easy to use, and fun. Dr. Yoshiro Hatano of Japan began studying pedometer use in the 1960s. He noted that Japanese adults who walked 10,000 steps per day had less stored fat, compared with those who walked less. Similar relationships have been shown in the United States. One study found that women who took at least 10,000 steps per day were in the normal weight range and weighed considerably less that women who averaged 6,000 to 10,000 steps per day (Fenton, 2006,), (Sidman, 2004). Recent research led by Dr. Lawrence Frank (2013) at the University of Vancouver British Columbia found that the risk of obesity rises six percent with each additional hour per day spent in a car. Another study (Cedric, 2003) concludes that watching two or more hours of television a day increases the risk of diabetes by more than ten percent and of obesity by nearly twenty-five percent. The pedometer is just the tool to help us be aware of how much we are sitting versus stepping.

Leroy (29) and Belle (27), a husband and wife, are not very active in their everyday life. They work together in the same office, they

---

1 More on that matter: President's Council on Physical Fitness and Sports: www.fitness.gov. The President's Council Active Lifestyle Program began in 2002 and encourages people to get active by doing 30 minutes of physical activity a day, five days for at least six weeks. Blue Cross/Blue Shields sponsors a WalkingWorks program at www.walkingworks.com to encourage Americans to get active. As one of the nation's largest health insurance providers, BCBS has a vested interest in keeping its members healthy and fit. Pedometers can be purchased at a very low price, and participants are encouraged to strive for 10,000 steps or 30 minutes of activity per day on five or more days a week. (Fenton, 2006).

mostly sit in comfortable office chairs every day, most of the day. An hour of Gymind training session once a week is not enough, so a recommendation to purchase a pedometer as a motivator for walking was almost inevitable. It was easier for Leroy. He simply took the dogs for longer walks each day (a win-win situation for both Leroy and the dogs). For Belle it was more of a challenge. She wrote me one night that she could not achieve her goal of 10,000 steps so she walked back and forth in front of the television only to be able to show me a "good number".

10,000 steps per day: For weight control and a healthier heart.

12,000 -15,000: For long-term health and a more noticeable weight loss.

3,000 of daily steps at a fast pace several days a week, to boost aerobic fitness. (Fenton, 2006).

Tami, a 12-year-old girl, was sent to me by her pediatrician more than a year ago. "The girl is not active, she hates sports", said her mom, distressed. "We eat very healthy at home, yet Tami is still overweight". Tami and I bonded instantly. I suggested she use a pedometer in order to take charge of her steps and movement. Since Tami's father travels often, and on one of his trips, he brought her an expensive "cool" pedometer. Not a day goes by without Tami sending me a picture of the number of steps she has taken. The goal: To maintain a minimum of 10,000 steps and exceed that number, if possible. From a "sports hater" as her mom described her, Tami became much more active and enthusiastic. "Look how high she can jump now", her mom bragged on one occasion. That's what it's all about, encouraging Tami to be more active and improve her everyday skills, jumping included.

Special shoes for walking? Oh yes!

Gabrielle was a dear client of mine back in 2008 when we lived in California. Gabrielle asked me just to come to her house three times per week and "walk her"." Yes, she laughed, just like you walk a dog". She worked long hours in her house and needed a personal trainer to motivate her into walking in the hope of easing chronic pains in her legs and feet that had been bothering her for years. Gabrielle also consulted a well-known chiropractor in the Bay-Area named Dave. She often talked about our personal sessions when she visited Dave; she often talked about Dave while walking with me. So that one day it was almost inevitable for us all to conduct a professional group meeting, Dave-Gabrielle-Myself, in order to discuss Gabrielle's health. One burning question I had for Dave, a question that had been in my mind for years, since way back during my BA studies when we learned how Ethiopians walk, and especially run, without shoes. "Dave, I asked: How important are shoes?" He looked at me astonished and somewhat disappointed and said: "VERY!"

1. Choose a shoe that bends easily through the ball of the foot but is fairly firm and won't bend easily through the arch.

2. A low heel is important. Don't pick a running shoe with big thick cushioning in the heel. The extra material in the heel tends to force your toes to slap down too quickly and can lead to shin discomfort as you walk (Fenton, 2001).

5 simple moves are recommended because they target the muscles that do much of the work in walking:

Ankle circles: Stand on one foot and slowly flex that ankle through its full range of motion, making circles with the toes.

Leg swings : Stand on one leg and swing the other loosely from the hip, front to back.

Pelvic loops: Put hands on hips with knees gently bent, feet apart at shoulder-width. Keep body upright and make 10 slow continuous circles with hips.

Arm circles: Body position like the letter T, (arms wide open), 10-12 slow backwards circles with hands, starting small finish with large using the entire arm. Shake arms and repeat forward.

Hula-hoop jumps: Hopping in place on both feet, twist feet and lower body left and then right 20 times.

"Power-walk" for your health

"Power walk" is a robust and strong method of walking, a wonderful technique to take our walking experience to the next level. The secret is to simply shift from the typical "window-shopping stroll" to a more athletic gait and pace. It takes a little practice, since thinking about the movement is involved, but the calorie burnt, an average of 400 for an hour of power walk, really pays off. How to walk the power walk? Apparently go faster. However, it's not only that. When we power-walk and think of all the elements of that technique, we reprogram the brain and the body, which is already used to a certain pattern of walking. So it becomes a "mind-walk" along with a "power walk" (Jordan, 2013).

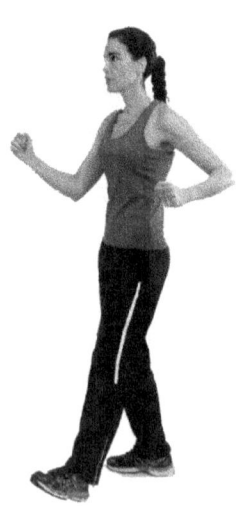

Pump your arms, driving your elbow straight back as you push your opposite hand forward. You bend your elbows to 90 degrees and swing your arms at your sides in opposition to your legs. That's the way to walk faster and maintain balance; this motion also works your upper body by strengthening your triceps and trunk.

Keep your stride a bit smaller than your natural stride length; simply take more steps in a shorter amount of time. Push off the ground through the ball of your foot, propelling yourself forward. That's the way to protect your back.

Keep your shoulders relaxed, maintain an upright posture and push off through your foot, thinking about your leg muscles with each step. That's the way to walk fast (Archer, 2010).

Walk and run backwards

It may feel awkward and inconvenient at first, but integrating walking and running backwards during your aerobic session can be freshening and most effective. A research from Medical College of Ohio confirmed that walking backward may place additional muscular demands on an individual (Cipriani, 1995). Concentric muscle activity in forward walking would become eccentric activity in backward walking, and vice versa. (Winter, 1989). Another study from the Institute and Faculty of Physical Therapy Taipei, Taiwan, demonstrated that asymmetric gait pattern in post-stroke patients could be improved from receiving additional backward walking therapy (Yang, 2005). This is a perfect way to work on your coordination, and improve balance and stability.

It's important to walk or run backwards in a safe environment such as a round stadium or a wide hall. You can peek backwards from time to time to regain confidence about your movement and direction.

5 minutes warm-up	Fast walk forward
2 minutes	Light jogging forward
5 minutes	Fast walk backwards
2 minutes	Light jogging backwards
5 minutes	Fast walk forward
2 minutes	Fast walk backwards You can retake this circuit 2-3 times in a row.

The spiritual side of walking (or running)

When we walk, we automatically move our feet, legs, and pelvis, our lower part of our body, our lower chakra. The "roots", not necessarily in the sense of our ancestors, (the collective), but our personal roots, "Because Man is a Tree of the Field" as wrote Nathan Zach, an Israeli poet. The Chakras are energetic centers in the body that are crucial to the flow of life force energy throughout our being. The balance and health of our chakras can determine the health and balance of our body. When these energetic centers are blocked or unbalanced, the flow of energy through the meridians of the body is disrupted, which can result in poor health, depression, and a general feeling of fatigue. (Ahsian, 1995). The word "Chakra" derives from the Sanskrit word for "wheel" or "turning", and they correspond to vital points in the physical body. The seven chakras system has become quite popular in the West since 1927.

The root chakra, (Muladhara), is located at the base of the spine in the coccygeal region. It's responsible for the fight-or-flight response when survival is under threat. Muladhara is related to instinct, security, survival and also to basic human potentiality. Physically, it governs sexuality; mentally it governs stability; emotionally it governs sensuality; spiritually it governs a sense of security.

The function of the chakras is to spin and draw in the energy of life, hence to keep the spiritual, mental, emotional and physical health of the body in balance. So that when we walk and move our body, we are basically reconnected to all of our qualities and characteristics; we open lines of energy and flow. When we decide to embrace walking as part of our everyday routine, we enjoy, even without being aware of it, the advantages of an open lower chakra and a better flow and balance between all seven chakras, since they all take an active part in walking.

Meet Barak on his "run" for happiness

One of the great advantages of walking or running is that those are physical activities that are almost always available. We are independent; we do not rely on the gym to be opened or on a friend to play tennis with. We are on our own, taking responsibility, taking charge. According to the Gymind way, it's almost impossible to separate the physical from the mental; this means, for example, that the ability to take responsibility is a pattern, a Gestalt that exists inside the person so that he is capable of taking charge of his body as well as of his mind. So that when the person makes a change in the physical part, change of the mental will not take long to appear.

Barak is a 28-year-old acupuncturist, recently graduated from college, taking his first steps as a therapist; inexperienced and with somewhat low self-esteem and inhibitions in executing his wishes and abilities. This is one level we discussed during sessions. The main reason Barak decided to delve deep in his soul was his relationship with his wife. He did not know how to put things into words, but he FELT something was not right. Barak felt his love life went downhill without his having any control of it. His wife, 6 years older than he is, (a sweet intelligent women, like her husband she is a therapist and an acupuncturist), was talking about the next step in their mutual life: Becoming parents. Barak was petrified; he felt as if he had to make a decision whether to stay married and have a baby, or break up and walk away.

The first thing he had to do was to regain a sense of control over his life. The writing was on the wall: Barak had always been taken with jogging. He used to jog years ago back in college but as the years went by, he gradually stopped. "I feel alive when I run" he confessed, "I know my allergies disappear, that I become stronger in body and spirit".

Integrating a jogging session in his schedule required him to rearrange his timetable and reorganize his choices in his everyday life.

Barak's training program

The main important component of Barak's training sessions was the Run. More than power exercises, strengthening the core or working on stretching and flexibility. They are all very important. But for him to start feeling really good about himself, which was the main key for regaining control and getting some answers about his love life, directing Barak to a daily routine that consisted of running - was crucial. I asked him to send me via email his vision of a good organized active timetable, one that would make him get up from bed with a smile or at least with a sense of "DOING" that would let him feel alive, active, healthy. Barak could easily start the day with a good run, so he said, and sent me that detailed email on March 10th 2013:

Sun	Mon	Tue	Wed	Thurs	Fri	Sat
10:30-11:00 jogging	10:30-11:00 jogging	10:30-11:00 jogging	Begins late after a night shift	10:30-11:00 jogging	Free time	Journey
12:00-14:00 Studying, writing	12:00-14:00 Studying and writing	12:00-14:00 Studying, writing		12:00-14:00 Studying and writing		
14-15 receiving patients	Work till 22:00	14-15 receiving patients		Work till 22:00		
15:00 cooking		15:00 cooking	-15:00 16:00 reading			
16:00-18:00 receiving patients plus T'ai Chi training		16:00-18:00 receiving patients plus T'ai Chi training	16:00-16:30 Riding bicycles			
18:00-18:30 playing guitar		18:00-18:30 playing guitar	21:00 Chinese			
21:00-22:00		21:00-22:00				

Meet Maya and the way to overcome a heart condition

Engaging in a serious cardio-vascular activity was a must for Maya, (29, engineer, married), according to her cardiologist.

Our first encounter took place on May 27th 2010, when Maya revealed her main goal: To enable her heart and her body to carry a baby through all nine months of pregnancy. A close and careful study of her medical file revealed several terminologies such as: Tetralogy of Fallot syndrome, a defect in the structure of the heart and great vessels, (present at Maya's birth), PPCMP: Peripartum

Cardiomyopathy, a rare and frequently reversible cause of heart failure, (present later on during Maya's pregnancy and delivery), and long RP SVT: Supraventricular Tachycardia.

Tetralogy of Fallot results in low oxygenation of blood due to the mixing of oxygenated and deoxygenated blood in the left ventricle via the VSD, (Venticular Septal Defect), and preferential flow of the mixed blood from both ventricles through the aorta because of the barrier to flow through the pulmonary valve; an inadequate flow of blood to the lungs for oxygenation, (right-to-left shunt). The mortality rate in untreated patients reaches 50% by age 6 but in the present era of cardiac surgery, children with simple forms of tetralogy of Fallot enjoy good long-term survival with an excellent quality of life (Shabir, 2013). So at the age of 9 months, on February 15th 1984, Maya underwent a "total anomalous venous return to coronary sinus" surgery.

26 years later and Maya's cardiologist advised her to get into shape before getting pregnant, in order to be able to safely carry her pregnancy. That was our main goal, so that the whole Gymind process was put together to achieve that goal, fitness-wise, nutrition-wise and what later on was revealed to be the most meaningful: Mind and Spirit wise.

Maya's training program

Walking, running, step-aerobics, cycle training, intervals, it was all there twice a week for an hour of aerobic work-out. The first several months of training revolved almost only around the cardio-vascular endurance. A Polar watch was a must so that we could monitor the pulse and work-out with extra caution: Not to overload, not to exaggerate. In order to "get Maya's heart in shape", any aerobic activity counted.

This example of a strong and vigorous training session enabled Maya to work on her cardiovascular endurance, (the heart's ability to deliver blood to working muscles and their ability to use it), while her pulse increases up to 85% of its maximum capacity for 10 minutes or even less (BrianMac, 2013):

Begin with a short dynamic warm-up in order to prepare joints and muscles, a 2 minute-walk will do the trick. You can perform one round of exercises 1-5, take 1 minute rest and go again for a second round.

Exercise no. 1: Jumping Jacks

Starting position: Stand with knees slightly bent and arms resting to the sides of your body.

Jump so that your legs are more than shoulder-width apart, extend arms and lift them above your head so that the palms touch. Go back to starting position.

How many? 10 repetitions, 3 sets, a 10 seconds rest between sets.

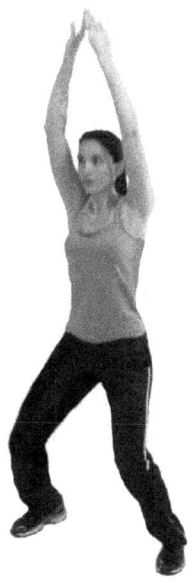

Exercise no. 2: Heels to your Glutes

Starting position: Stand with legs more than shoulder-width apart; extend arms in front of your body on shoulders level.

Lean forward, jump high and bring your left heels to your glutes. Change to the right leg while jumping.

How many? 20 repetitions, 3 sets, a 10 seconds rest between sets.

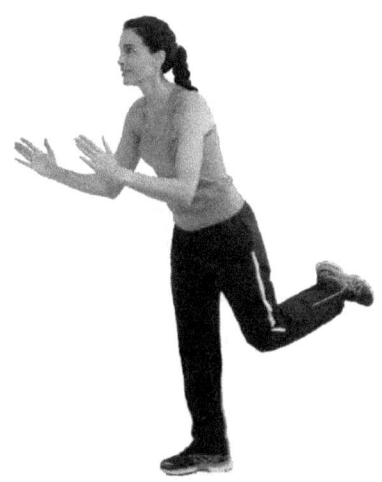

Exercise no. 3: Sides jumping

Starting position: Stand with knees slightly bent and arms resting to the sides of your body.

Jump with both legs from side to side. Keep your knees slightly bent on landing and keep your abs strong and core muscles tucked in. In order to raise the bar, you can jump higher and longer distances.

How many? 20 repetitions, 2 sets, a 10 seconds rest between sets.

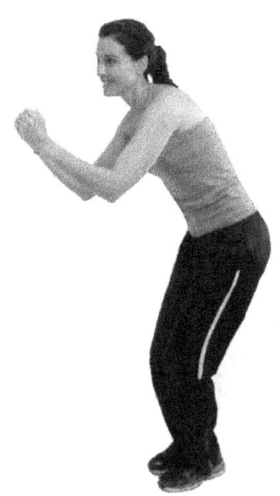

Exercise no. 4: On the step

Starting position: Stand behind the step with your knees slightly bent legs more than shoulder-width apart.

Jump on the step with both legs. Keep your knees slightly bent on landing and keep your abs strong and core muscles tucked in.

Gently go back to position number 1, without jumping.

How many? 10 repetitions, 3 sets, a 10 seconds rest between sets.

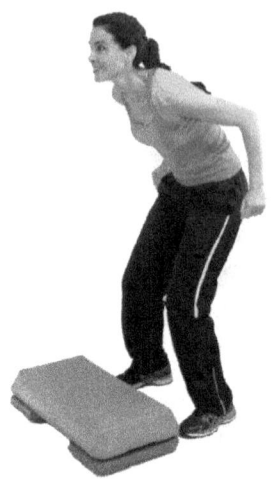

Exercise no. 5: Don't skip your skipping rope

Starting position: Hold your rope in front of your body just before beginning to jump.

Jump, skip, as you use one leg after the other.

How many? Two minutes in a row.

The anaerobic cycle training

This would be an example of an anaerobic training session in order to strengthen Maya's core, obtain optimal mobility and physical strength.

Exercise no. 1: Walk with Power
Works on: Preparing muscles and joints for the activity, strengthens arms and thighs.

Starting position: Stand up comfortably and hold a power ball or a 4 lb. weight in your hands.

Step back and forth while lifting up your knees; swing your arms up to a 90 degrees angle in an opposite direction to the leg you lift.

How many? 8 steps forwards, 8 steps backwards, 5 times in a row.

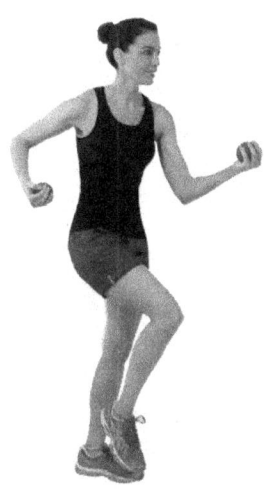

Exercise no. 2: For arms and thighs
Works on: Pectoralis major (chest), scapulas, thighs, glutes, coordination.

Starting position: Stand up comfortably and hold a power ball or a 4 Lb. weight in your hands, arms bent in front of your chest as shown.

Open your elbows (bring your scapulas closer) and lift your right leg to the side.

How many? 8 lifts of the right leg, 8 lifts of the left leg, 6 right, 6 left, 4 right 4 left 2 right 2 left then one after the other 8 times in a row.

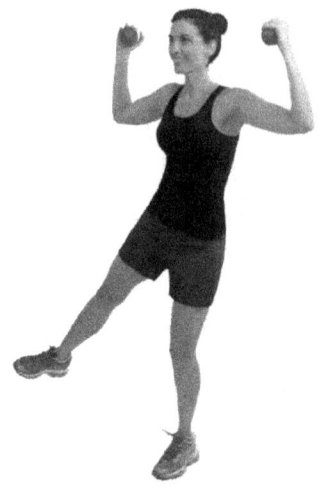

Exercise no. 3: Bowling with Balance
Works on: Arms, thighs, glutes, balance and coordination.

Starting position: Stand in a step-forward-position, each hand holds a weight.

Make a bowling move with right arm (as if you are about to toss the weight) and lean forward while lifting the right leg up. Work slowly.

How many? 10 lifts with right side, 10 with left, 3 sets in a row.

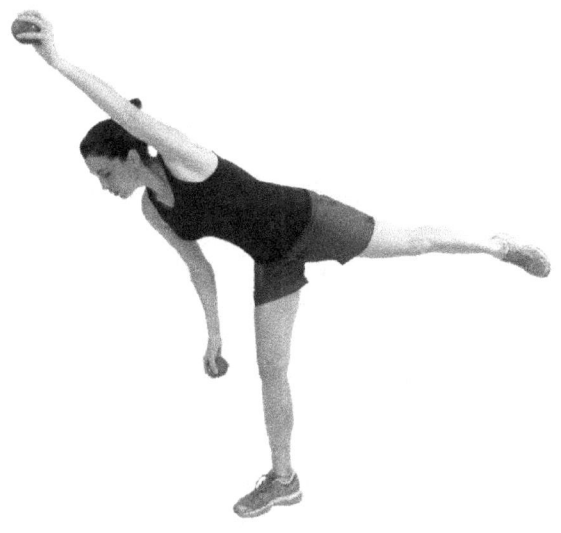

Exercise no. 4: Squat with a cross
Works on: Arms, thighs, glutes, chest.

Starting position: Stand up, knees slightly bent, hold a weight on each arm.

Take a squat to your right and place both arms crossed in front of your chest. Go back to position 1.

How many? 10 squats to your right, 10 to your left. 2 sets, a 15-sec rest between sets.

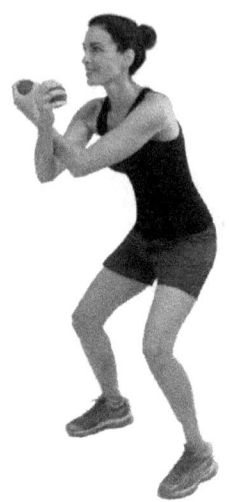

Exercise no.5: Diagonal weights
Works on: Arms, shoulders, abdominals.

Starting position: Lie down on your back with your knees bent and feet on the ground. Each arm holds the weight; right arm reaches toward the ceiling, as shown.

Bring your knees to your right and move the right arm toward your left side above and over the body. Hold position for two seconds.

How many? 15 repetitions to your left, 15 to your right, 2 sets in a row.

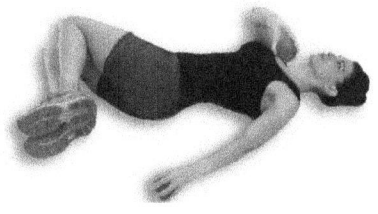

Exercise no.6: Half a bridge
Works on: Arms, abdominals, glutes, balance, coordination.

Starting position: Lie down on your back with your knees bent and feet on the ground. Each arm holds the weight and placed to the side of your body.

Lift your left leg straight to the ceiling. Squeeze your glutes and keep your abs tucked in. Raise your arms up towards the ceiling without "locking" your elbows.

How many? 8 times with your left leg, 8 with your right, 3 sets, 10 seconds rest between sets.

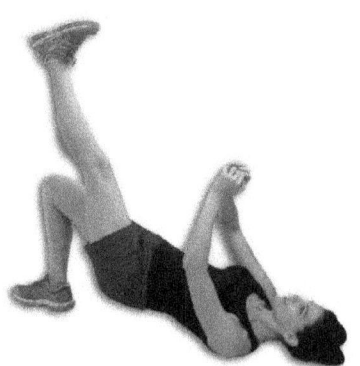

Children's activity

In a world where technology dominates, children seem to be spending less time playing outdoors than ever before. According to the American Heart Association, (2013), inactive children are likely to become inactive adults. Encouraging the development of physical activity habits in children helps establish patterns that continue into adulthood. Childhood obesity has reached epidemic proportions worldwide and is associated with increased cardiovascular mortality and morbidity in adult life (Watts, 2005). The vast majority of scientific evidence supports the beneficial role of exercise in achieving body weight stability and overall health (Chaput, 2011).

Obesity rates in the United States have reached epidemic proportions: 58 million overweight; 40 million obese; Eight out of 10 adults over age 25 overweight; 78% of American's do not meet basic activity level recommendations; 25% completely sedentary; 76%

increase in Type II diabetes in adults 30-40 yrs. old since 1990; In 2001 25% of all white children and 33% of African American and Hispanic children were overweight. According to the Centers for Disease Control and Prevention, 16 percent of children (over 9 million) 6-19 years old are overweight or obese, a number that has tripled since 1980. In addition to the 16 percent of children and teens ages 6 to 19 who were overweight in 1999-2002, another 15 percent were considered at risk of becoming overweight. According to the Centers for Disease Control and Prevention, (2004), over the past three decades the childhood obesity rate has more than doubled for preschool children aged 2-5 years and adolescents aged 12-19 years, and it has more than tripled for children aged 6-11 years.

Findings of a study managed at the Brown University Medical School demonstrate a number of differences in children's eating and activity habits on weekends and weekdays. They also suggest that attending to differences in food intake and activity habits on weekdays and weekends separately may help to identify periods of high risk, which could be modified with effective intervention approaches (Hart, 2011).

The increase in fat mass in children and adolescents has occurred concomitantly with a decline in reported time for exercise. According to several studies (Watts, 2005) held at the School of Human Movement and Exercise Science, the University of Western Australia, it has been suggested that prevention of obesity in childhood and adolescence should emphasize increased physical activity rather than diet because of fears relating to the adverse effects of inappropriate eating patterns. These studies indicate that although exercise training does not consistently decrease bodyweight or body mass index, it is associated with beneficial changes in fat and lean body mass.

All children, even less-coordinated, need to be physically active. Activity may be particularly helpful for the physical and psychological well-being of children with a weight problem. School-age youth should participate daily in 60 minutes or more of moderate to vigorous physical activity that is developmentally appropriate, enjoyable, and involves a variety of activities. (Strong, 2005). When most adults think about exercise, they imagine working out in the gym on a treadmill or lifting weights. But for kids, exercise means playing and being physically active. Kids exercise when they have gym class at school, during recess, at dance class or soccer practice, while riding bikes, or when playing tag. Besides enjoying the health benefits of regular exercise, kids who are physically fit sleep better and are better able to handle physical and emotional challenges, from running to catch a bus to studying for a test. (Numerous.org). A recent study held at the Department of Kinesiology and Community Health, University of Illinois at Urbana-Champaign, (Pontifex, 2013), indicates that even single bouts of moderately intense aerobic exercise may have positive implications for aspects of neurocognitive function and inhibitory control in children with ADHD. Another study held in Department of Physical Therapy, Lebanon Valley College, Annville, Pennsylvania, (Oriel, 2011), showed noticeably how aerobic exercise prior to classroom activities may improve academic response in young children with autism spectrum disorder.

According to a study held at the Faculty of Physical Education and Physiotherapy, Department of Human Biometry and Biomechanics at the University of Brussels, because regular physical activity of high enough intensity is essential in the management of overweight, efforts should be made to increase adherence to physical activity in overweight children. To motivate overweight children to exercise and follow the recommendations, it is essential to create opportunities to satisfy the need for autonomy, (having choices), competence, (feeling effective) and relatedness, (being socially connected). To increase feelings of autonomy in overweight children, exercise programs could be delivered in an autonomy-supportive manner by providing choices, supporting the child's initiatives, avoiding use of external rewards, offering relevant information and rationale for changing behavior, while minimizing pressure and control. Feelings of relatedness in overweight children might increase by adopting an empathic approach, showing interest in the child's well-being and problems, showing enjoyment and enthusiasm, knowing the names of the children, talking to the children as equals, offering group sessions and talks, encouraging club participation and having a sports partner, and encouraging parental support. (Deforche, 2011).

The American Heart Association recommends:

Physical activity should be increased by reducing sedentary time (watching television, playing computer video games, or talking on the phone).

Physical activity should be fun for children and adolescents.

Parents should try to be role models for active lifestyles and provide children with opportunities for increased physical activity.

Children age 2 and older should participate in at least 60 minutes of enjoyable, moderate-intensity physical activities every day that are developmentally appropriate and varied.

If your child or children don't have a full 60-minute activity break each day, try to provide at least two 30 minute periods or four 15 minutes periods in which they can engage in vigorous activities appropriate to their age, gender, and stage of physical and emotional development.

Meet Oliver and the needs of a 12-year-old boy

Oliver and I first met on November 11th 2010 when he was 12 years old, 140 cm, 62 kg, a sweet "chubby" charming, articulate, smart, and captivating young man. A real "rainbow kid" [2] with a great soul, sensitivity, and intuition.

Oliver's goals:

---

2 The term "rainbow kid" will be discussed in chapter 3.

Losing weight

Getting in shape

Making a change in life (his words)

Enjoy social acceptance.

Oliver is the youngest of three brothers. His mom is an art teacher and his dad an organizational consultant; he is a beautiful boy born to a loving family from a rural settlement in the center of Israel.

Oliver experienced some difficulties in facing the world. He was diagnosed at the age of three (and again at four and at five years old) as "immature, maladroit, and awkward", both in speech and movement (February 2003). He had several deficiencies and weaknesses that prevented him from fitting in and being like everybody else.

According to a psychological report, (2004), based on:

Oliver's preschool teacher recommendations, (February 26th 2003).

The preschool psychologist, (February 2003),

Child development center, (March, July 2003) and the Occupational Therapist's report (May-June 2003).

Oliver came into the world after a rough pregnancy and a difficult delivery. His motoric development was slow in comparison to other children and to his brothers at the same age. In other areas, his development was normal and his interaction with other children was good. However, he had some difficulties in organizing a sentence, in expressing himself; he avoided certain games and dealing with unfamiliar tasks. This led to frustrations and childish reactions inappropriate to his age. According to the psychologist's report, (2004), Oliver's weaknesses were somewhat minor but enough to impede his normal development and to make it hard for him to fit in.

The psychologist's recommendations were: Oliver must continue to learn in a small protective setting or in a normal preschool with a personal assistant (shadow) to help him get fit. Oliver should work with a speech therapist, a motoric therapist, and with his parents to enable him to face difficulties in life.

Mom as a rescuer, a mediator to the world

Oliver's father received the troubling news about Oliver's difficulties with resignation. However, Oliver's mom did not give up and together they fought for Oliver to have a brighter future. This is a child with an "inner world", whose speech is constructed by associations. Oliver's mom tells that he had a habit of talking to his hands as if they were puppets, creating his own world, almost shutting himself off from others or protecting himself from an intimidating world. At the age of four Oliver had almost reached his goals. The recommendations were for him to stay one more year at that special preschool. His mom insisted that the pedagogical board reconsider the decision several months later, (so as not to lose another school year), and gradually helped Oliver integrate in a regular setting: one day at a regular preschool, then two days, until within six month, at the age of five Oliver was ready to interact full time with regular kids in a regular school.

The special education also had a vital social benefit: it enabled Oliver's mom to do the "social work" outside of school and to organize social interactions with neighbors and friends in the afternoons.

Oliver suffers from a condition in his heart at the form of Premature ventricular contractions (PVCs): early, extra heartbeats that originate in the ventricles. Most of the time, PVCs don't cause any symptoms or require treatment, (Lindsay, 2013), and so we could "dive into the deep water" and exercise without further delay.

Oliver's medical history

Diagnosed in early infancy as hypotonic, Oliver needs to strengthen his muscle tone. Hypotonia is a state of low muscle tone or muscle strength. It is not a specific medical disorder, (Goldenring, 2011), but a potential manifestation of different disorders that affect motor nerve control by the brain or muscle strength. Diagnosing the underlying cause is often unsuccessful, but treatment such as physical therapy, occupational therapy yields positive results.

For instance, infants with normal tone can be lifted with the parent's hands placed under their armpits. Hypotonic infants tend to slip between the hands as the infant's arms rise without resistance. With Oliver. at the age of 12, the hypotonia was clear and evident, for example, when he was jumping on the grand trampoline. Jumping up and down made Oliver's arms (which seemed "loose" and "stress-free") to be "all over the place" putting both shoulders at risk of being dislocated.

Prior to our work together, he had undergone hydrotherapy treatment for two years, three years of gymnastics, art therapy, swimming lessons, (until the age of 11), and tennis class in a small group. Still, Oliver needed to regain control over his movements, his muscles, and his body.

Oliver was enthusiastic to begin. Anxious and worried about the future as he seemed to be, there was still a spirited look in his eyes. He was ready to begin.

"I need a CHANGE" was a phrase repeated during our first encounter session. His will-power was so strong that every physical challenge I gave him – whether it was a certain jump on the trampoline or a balance routine on the balance board – was accepted with joy and excitement, no matter how tough the assignments were for him. The 12 year-old was perfectly clear about his goal in life, and I was captivated by his will-power and inner strength, strength it would take some time to build physically.

Oliver's physical training

Oliver was instructed to be more active in his every-day life. To ride his bicycle more often, to walk over to friend's house, to take a walk to the boy's scouts sessions. To be aware of the fact that he is more active and to give himself full credit for it.

Oliver used to play tennis twice a week. When he gave up on tennis, he went to swim class twice a week. Oliver was encouraged to participate in any sports activity he wishes .

We meet once a week at the studio, practicing cardio-vascular training for 15 min:

Trampoline

Jogging

Kick-boxing

Cycle training

Strength training for 5-10 minutes:

Total-Gym

TRX

Light weights and 4 Lb. power balls

Functional exercises with bands, fit-balls, steps

Coordination and balance:

Balance board, Bossu

Basketball

Weeks went by, and Oliver started to lose weight rapidly. With his new nutrition plan and Mind therapy, Oliver blossomed.

Meet Liana and the needs of this 4- year-old girl

The vast majority of scientific evidence supports a beneficial role of exercise on achieving body weight stability and overall health, for children (future adults). The goal is to find ways to motivate them to exercise and adopt healthy lifestyles. In order to achieve this objective, we must be innovative and creative in finding ways to fight against the modern way of living that drives excess energy intake relative to expenditure. (Booth, 2000). A study held in The Exercise Physiology Laboratory, Bloomsburg University of Pennsylvania, aimed to determine the maximal cardiorespiratory responses of 48, 5- to 6 year old children (24 girls and 24 boys), who were tested on a treadmill and on an electronically-braked cycle ergometer. It was not surprising that all children improved their physiological criteria. (LeMura, 2001).

Liana detests the treadmill. I once was compelled to hold her for a whole 4 minutes in order to keep her on it, convincing, cheering, while she was stomping on the treadmill reluctant and even resentful. The process of physical activity with Liana was by far more challenging than with any other kid I have encountered.

At the age of 4, (on our first encounter, November 4th 2012), Liana was 110 cm, weighing 31.6 with a BMI of 26, way up in the chart as far as child obesity is concerned. Exercising with her was fun at first: Running around all over the studio, getting acquainted with fun-fitness-prompts such as the fit-ball or the jumping rope. Liana enjoyed a good sweat, feeling her body, enjoying using it. However, it was not always the case. When things became tougher, Liana gave up almost instantly, wishing to stay in her "comfort zone". The trampoline was a huge challenge. Liana could not bear the thought of disconnecting her feet from solid ground. She dreaded the moment. So I held both her hands, but even then she jumped leaning forward since her belly would not let her jump straight up. Same thing with the treadmill. For 30 seconds it was fun. Longer than that? Her small feet had a hard time carrying her body so that for her it was hard. Heavy. Burning. Repetitious.

Things did not progress as I anticipated. Liana was active one a week at my studio but preferred drawing or spending long afternoons in front of the TV watching her favorite "Dora the Explorer" shows at home.

We had to integrate physical activities with her sedentary behavior and make her "move" more during the day. One of the major problems was that Liana did not understand WHY she needed to sweat. It was so much easier and nicer to just sit, chat, or draw. If the trampoline is a problem, for example, the easiest thing would be to avoid it. To avoid the treadmill. To ignore what is so difficult and continue as usual without interruption. She protested against coming to my studio so that her parents began to bribe her with candies to agree to show up for a session. What a surreal picture it was: Liana with a big bag of potato chips in one hand, a large box of chocolate in the other, wearing a forced smile and walking down the stairs to begin a training session.

Engaging the family in the Gymind process

The family's involvement was a crucial step for us. Liana's parents were told right from the start that without a holistic change at home, as far as nutrition and physical activities, a significant change would be out of reach. One cannot expect a 4-year-old child to make an effort while the family just watches, doing practically nothing. A study held at the Department of Nutrition Sciences, School of Health Related Professions, emphasized how important schools, families, and communities are as far as preventing childhood obesity. (Goran, 1999). According to Epstein, a leading authority on childhood obesity and professor of pediatrics at the University at Buffalo, (2013), when parents make healthy eating and being more physically active a family priority, they don't treat their overweight children differently than the rest of the family, (Liana has two older brothers), by placing them on diets or exercise programs outside of the regular family routine, a strategy that typically produces only minimal, short-term results. Including all family members in the behavior-change effort will benefit the health of all family members, even if they are not obese.

Liana, like any young child, closely models her parents. So several changes were made at home:

No more eating in front of the TV set. It leads to consuming more unhealthy food and eating more calories.

No more stocking the kitchen cabinets with junk food.

The TV set, the focus of family life, creates a sedentary environment that is unhealthy. No more. Now, when Liana's family gathers around to sit and watch TV, they now do it while sitting on a giant fit-ball so that muscles and balance work is constantly there.

Daily family walks that add physical activity to the family lifestyle, walks they often take to the park and have great fun as a family.

Liana does not carry by herself all that pressure to be active and lose the weight. She has her family physical and moral support. It has been several months now that Liana is training with her mom at my studio and both brothers and the Liana's father are training together on a different day of the week. A pedometer was brought to the house and I get a lot of family pictures during the week-ends showing how active they all are taking long walks, climbing mountains or riding their bikes.

Working-out according to your age; recommended fitness plan

The way we age is determined by more than just our DNA. Mounting evidence suggest that exercise can help delay and even reverse aging's debilitating effects on muscles, heart and brain. (Mc

Quaide-Little, 2012). Exercise, according to the National Institute of Aging (NIA, 20112), may even forestall the disabilities and diseases which were previously thought of as the unavoidable price of growing old. Even if exercise is initiated late in life, it can still delay the effects of aging, as we will see later in this chapter. A plan for our 20s, 30s 40s and 50s can shed a light on the physiological shifts the body goes through and develop an important awareness about our muscles, abilities and strength.

20s-30s: Power and Agility

As a young man, you are at the prime of your physiological abilities. You can very easily increase muscle tone, enjoy optimal functionality of the nervous system as far as responsiveness and agility, your balance and coordination and even your metabolic rate at rest is at its highest level. You can and may feel the need to perform high intensity activities, almost every day. Go for it. You are physiology in your top, enjoying a strong muscle tone and a perfect ability to execute intense, frequent exercise may it be aerobic or anaerobic. The reason for that ability would be a high level of human growth hormone (HGH) and testosterone currents that spur growth of the muscle fibers that ignite explosive lifts, sprints, jumps, and swings. (Brant, 2010). A recent research from the University of Florida, Department of Aging and Geriatric confirm that man's HGH levels drop from 6 nanograms per milliliter (ng/ml) when he's 20 to 3 ng/ml when he's 40, and that young man react much better for resistance training than older man. (Sinha-Hikim, 2002), (Manini, 2012).

Your 20s represent the best time to build muscular power, which consists of generating maximum force as quickly as possible. To exploit this moment, you can head straight for the heavy weights.

Although take notice: On average, the guys chose bodies with 30 pounds more muscle. By contrast, when women were asked to select men's bodies they found attractive, they chose guys with 15 to 30 pounds less muscle than the male participants had selected. (Oliverdia, 2005).

Exercises for the 20-30 year old man:

Squats with weights

Starting position: Your legs spread apart, knees slightly bent, each hand holds a 3 kg weight.

Preform a deep squat position while lifting both arms over your head. Go back to starting position.

How many? 10 squats, 3 sets, a 15 sec. rest between sets.

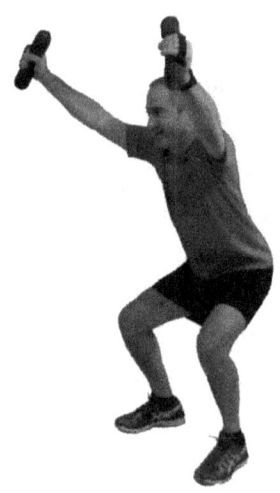

Classic push-ups

Starting position: Push-up position, keep your abs tucked-in and your head in alignment with your back.

Bend your elbows and lift one leg straight up.

How many? 10-15 repetitions with your right leg lifted, 10-15 repetitions with your left leg lifted, a 30 sec. rest between two sets.

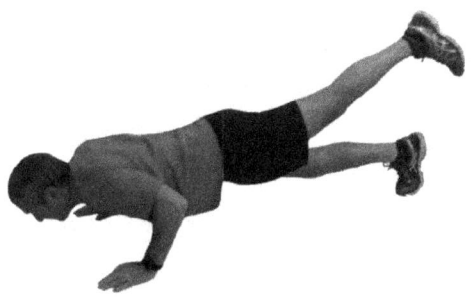

The Plyometric training or explosive moments is also suitable for you, since jumps allow strength to be converted to power. Jumps train mainly your nerves, while weights train your muscles. In fact, along with helping you gain speed and power, according to several studies, doing plyometric exercises also builds new muscle (Bompa, 2002), (Panton, 2004).

Put your strength to the test: The vertical jumping test

The vertical jumping test (Harman, 1991), is designed to measure the explosive strength of your *lower* limbs. All you need is a high wall, such as the outside of a building, and a bit of room so you can jump and land safely.

Start by standing side on to a wall and reach up as high as you can with the hand closest to the wall. Make note of how high you can reach. This is called the standing reach height. Then jump high as possible using both arms and legs to assist in projecting the body upwards. Measure the distance between the standing reach height and the maximum jump height, and that is your result.

rating	males (cm)	females (cm)
excellent	> 70	> 60
very good	61-70	51-60
above average	51-60	41-50
average	41-50	31-40
below average	31-40	21-30
poor	< 30	< 20

As a young woman, you are also in your prime for every physiological parameter. Your flexibility, your joints, your muscle strength, and your healthy bones allow you to be as sporty as you want, light and carefree. Your metabolism is 10 percent lower than that of men at your age, but as far as cardiovascular abilities and blood flow are concerned, you are on the top (McPhee, 2013). In your 20s your bone mass is at its best; you should keep it that way with proper nutrition and training programs to prevent it from deteriorating in the future (Teegarden, 1995).

Exercises for the 20-30 year-old woman

Rear push-up with one leg up

Starting position: Get down to a rear push-up position as shown.

Bend your elbows as you lift and straighten one leg up to the same level of the other knee.

How many? 10 repetitions with right leg, 10 repetitions with left leg,

30 seconds rest between sets.

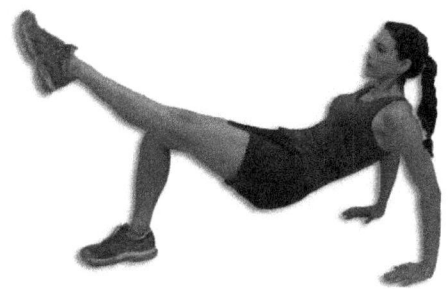

High Jumps

Starting position: Squat to jump.

Jump high and bring your knees to your chest.

How many? 7-10 consecutive jumps.

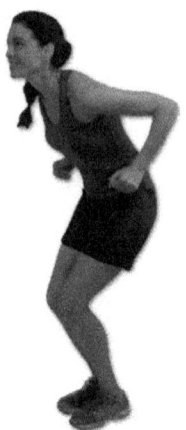

Your weekly training plan :(for man and women, 3 times a week):

15 minutes: aerobic training	40 minutes: Power training	5 minutes: stretching
2 min. warm-up of fast walk	Resistance training should include all the muscles in your body as shown earlier on in this chapter.	Make sure you stretch every muscle you worked on during your work-out.
5 min. light jogging (you can hold a conversation while jogging)	The way to build muscle strength would be to perform small amount of repetitions on a relatively heavy resistance, 65-85 % of RM1.	Stay still in stretching position for at least 10 seconds and breathe all the way through your stretch.
15 sprints of 15 sec. each, a 45 sec. walk for recovery between sprints	You can use machines on your local gym; attend a power class in a studio nearby, or embrace your own sets of exercises at home.	

Meet Muriel and the needs of this 22 year old girl

Muriel, 22, came to my studio on august 31st, 2009. I still hold on to that first email she wrote me a week prior for our encounter: "I am considered to be a pretty girl but so fat that nobody can tell..." And was she right. The first thing I noticed when first opened the door for her was two big eyes connected to a body, quite large one, no neck at sight. 158 cm weighing 93 kg. with a BMI of 37.3. Measurements: L Right arm 39 cm, Belly 101 cm., Right thigh 69 cm.

During our first session we went for a long walk-and-jog training and even though she had a difficult time performing (raising her pulse up to 180 BPM.), we saw the great potential of a motivated young girl with basic aerobic abilities. It was only the heavy weight of a high percentage of body fat that prevented her from running relatively easily.

A suitable and smart nutrition plan was a Must for this all-you-can-eat-junk-food-lover, crucial for her weight-loss process, and will be discussed in Chapter Two.

"My inner power drove me to success. I wanted to look good and to feel healthy," Muriel was quoted in Menta Magazine on September 2012 (weighting 58 kg and wearing a huge smile). She rarely missed a training session and she worked hard.

Muriel's training sample over a period of 3 months

30 minutes warm-up + cardio training	25 minutes resistance training + stretching	5 minute: relaxation and therapy.
First month: Interval training Kick boxing Power walk Step aerobic 93 kg 39,101,69.	Working on all muscles group with band, fit-ball and 2 kg weights.	Visualization and body image. For example: "Get into a full relaxation mode. Take three deep breathes and imagine a wide White screen in front of you. See your image in that screen: happy, healthy, thin, dynamic and complete. Make that picture as colorful as you wish, make it vivid and bright. Multiple those happy feeling 10 times more, 100 times more, a million times more. Now let that powerful image flow into your body. Feel that image absorbed inside every cell of your body".

Second month: Circuit training Step aerobics: advanced moves Basketball Elliptical 88 kg 35.5, 95, 65.	Working on all muscles group with 3 kg weights, higher resistance bands and power ball.	The swish pattern technique: To change a bad habit of the amount of food Muriel had consumed.
Third month: Jogging High intense interval training. 81.8 35,93,65	Working on all muscles group with 4 kg weights, total-gym cables. Later on we will use TRX for both aerobic and anaerobic trainings.	Energetic spiritual therapy, balancing chakras. Will be discussed on chapter 3.

30s-40s : Strength and Stamina

As a young man in your 30s, you encounter a slight decline from your physiological peak in your 20s: metabolic rate declines and body fat percentage may rise a notch. But if you exercise well, you can still be in the prime of your abilities (Nguyen, 1997). You can still extend your lactate threshold, the point when your muscles pump out fatigue-producing lactate faster than the blood can clear it and the muscles start burning more carbohydrates than fat. By extending your lactate threshold, you can exercise at a higher intensity, burn more calories, and better control your weight (Kraemer, 1998). This is the decade when you should keep your body fat percentage on less than 22, in order to avoid high blood pressure, diabetes, and heart disease. (Berset, 1992). The solution: Drink water; keep healthy snacks and fresh fruits in a bag and at your office desk to avoid fasting long hours which leads to extensive eating at dinner time. That's the way to maintain a healthy metabolism and an invigorated feeling during a hard day at work.

Exercises for the 30-40 year old men

Use a Fit-ball

Starting position: Place your abdominals on a fit-ball.

Spread your arms to the sides and raise your back as shown. Work slowly and maintain your head aligned with your back.

How many? 10 repetitions, 3 sets, a 30 sec. rest between sets.

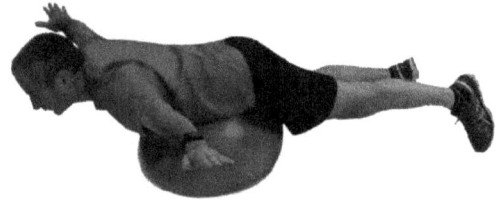

To your abs with fit-ball.

Starting position: Lie down on your back and place fit-bell between your thighs as shown.

Bring fit-ball to your chest and go back to starting position.

How many? 15 repetitions, 3 sets, a one minute rest between sets.

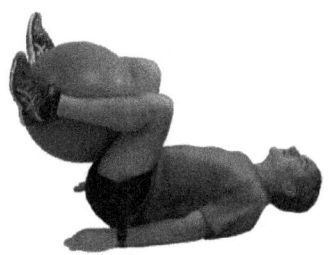

Your weekly work-out plan

25 minutes: aerobic interval training

A real short-cut on your way to a healthy, fit body, interval training is a compromise between time-consuming moderate-intensity training and sprint-interval training requiring all-out efforts. This intensive training allows you to work nearly half the time of your regular "flat" walk or run. (Perry, 2008). Here is an example of interval training on your treadmill.

Time (min.)	Speed (KMH)	Elevation (%)
5	6.6	0
2	10	0
5	7	2
2	7	6
5	10	0
2	6.5	6
3	6	8

25 minutes: strength training

The goal here is power endurance; hence, perform a relatively high number of repetitions on a relatively light weight, 50-60 percent of your potential RM1 (Repetition Maximum, the heaviest weight you can lift once). You can use machines at your local gym; attend a power class in a studio nearby, or adopt your own sets of exercises at home, working on all muscle groups.

10 minutes: stretching

At the end of your training session remember to stretch properly. Perform static stretches for every muscle and stay in position for at least 10 seconds. Remember to breathe throughout your stretch.

As a young woman at your 30s, maintaining an active life-style, performing resistance training and pursuing a smart diet with emphasis on calcium intake is important at this stage of your life to prevent osteoporosis in your near future. Towards the end of this decade, there may be a decline in estrogen hormones which may cause loss of muscle tissue (Nelson, 2008). While men experience a very gradual decline in testosterone which helps them maintain their bone density and muscle strength, it's an unfair advantage (Booth, 2010). A study from the Department of Health and Kinesiology, Texas A&M University confirms that high exercise intensities and endurance training elicits favorable oxygen uptake adaptations and help prevent estrogen decline (Green, 2002). During this decade you should work on two physical components: aerobic competence and strength. You may be a mom by now, and those abilities will help you be more vital when taking care of your kids.

Meet Irene and her fight against Lupus

Our first encounter occurred on January 3rd 2011. A 37-year-old woman, 162 cm, 68.5 kg, came to my studio, and I could hardly anticipate the long and profound journey we were about to embark on together. Irene was to embody every aspect of the Gymind way, both mentally and physically and she was ready for the hard work that was ahead. Irene felt she needed a mental support, (she was not sure she could stay married for one day longer), she needed to lose some weight, and most of all she had been diagnosed with Lupus, an autoimmune deficiency syndrome, several months prior to our encounter. Medications, as she put it, "were out of the question".

With each week of work Irene grew stronger in both body and soul; the mental and the physical parts of her being were hard to separate. When Irene strengthened her muscles, she simultaneously strengthened her soul, becoming more positive and passionate about life and goals. The mental process Irene went through will be discussed at length in Chapter 3 of this book.

Systemic lupus erythematosus is an autoimmune disease in which the body's immune system mistakenly attacks healthy tissues. It can affect the skin, joints, kidneys, brain, and other organs. The underlying cause of autoimmune diseases is not fully known. Lupus is much more common in women than men. It may occur at any age, but appears most often in people between the ages of 10 and 50 (Ruiz Irastorza, 2010). Over the past 4 decades, the incidence of Systemic lupus erythematosus has nearly tripled, and there has been a statistically significant improvement in survival. These findings are likely due to a combination of improved recognition of mild forms of the disease and better approaches to therapy (Uramoto, 1999).

The disease is characterized by a variety of symptoms, especially fatigue, pain, and reduced quality of life. Accumulating evidence indicates that regular exercise is beneficial in improving vascular function and disease-related symptoms associated with Systemic lupus erythematosus (Barnes, 2012), improving cardiovascular fitness, reducing metabolic abnormalities and fatigue, and improving quality of life (Ayan, 2007).

A study from the Department of Medicine at the University Medical School, Chicago found that patients in both exercise groups (aerobic and anaerobic) showed some improvement in fatigue, functional status, cardiovascular fitness and muscle strength. Both groups showed increased bone turnover, but bone mineral density was unchanged. (Ramsey-Goldman, 2000). A study from the National Sports Medicine Institute in London tested the efficacy of a graded aerobic exercise program in treating fatigue in systemic lupus erythematosus and supported the benefits of training on patients' overall feeling (Tench, 2003). Researches on that subject are numerous: Strombeck) 2007), Forte (1999), Carvalho (2005) and many more. All evidence of the effectiveness of physical training be it mild or moderate, aerobic or resistance training, they should all be conducted carefully for this population (Barnes, 2012). That's exactly what convinced Irene to begin a controlled exercise program. We did (and still do) it all: aerobic sessions, intervals with moderate or high intensities, kick-boxing, jogging, power trainings with weights, bands, TRX and power-balls with high resistance. Irene loves to feel her body; she enjoys the pain that comes from working hard as opposed to the pain the disease causes. In fact, Irene was so caught up with exercising, (mainly because it made her feel so good), that at the age of 39, two years into her Gymind process, she enrolled in the Zinman College of Physical Education at the Wingate Institute of Israel and after long exciting 9 months of studying, she became a certified trainer.

Exercises for the 30-40 year old woman

Chest Presses

Starting position: Stand with legs more than shoulder-width apart, knees slightly bent, and hold a fit-ball in front of your chest.

While jogging or walking on the spot, perform long and hard squeezes of the ball at chest level, higher than chest level and lower than chest level, alternately.

How many? 10 presses at chest level, 10 higher, 10 lower, 3 times in a row.

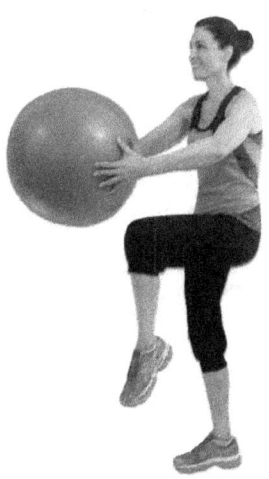

Thigh presses and lifts

Starting position: Sit down and lean on your palms. Place ball between your thighs.

Squeeze the ball with your thighs and bring your knees to your chest. Return to starting position.

How many? 10 presses, 10 lifts to chest, 3 times in a row.

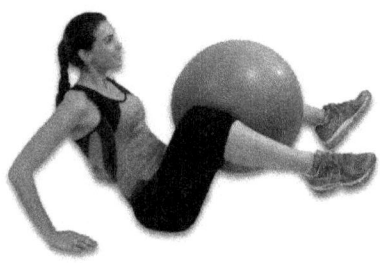

Your weekly work-out plan

25 minutes: Aerobic interval training

Time (min.)	Speed (KMH)	Elevation (%)
5	5	0
2	5.5	4
5	6	0
2	6.5	6
5	6.5	0
2	6.5	6
5	5.5	8

25 minutes: Strength training

Yoga or Pilates sessions are good for you. You may adopt your own sets of exercises at home, as long as you work on all muscle groups thoroughly and slowly, and remember to breathe.

10 minutes: Stretching

At the end of your training session, remember to stretch properly. Perform static stretches for every muscle and stay in position for a least 10 seconds. Remember to breathe throughout your stretch.

40s-50s : Flexibility and Strength

You are a man in your 40s, an age that marks the shift you make by starting to carry about your body at the gym instead of "punishing" it (Brant, 2010). If you have been taking care of yourself all through your 20s and 30s, you can easily feel the difference between your physical abilities and those of your friends who are out of shape as far as climbing the stairs or running a kilometer. Your nerve fibers are losing their effectiveness, which diminishes coordination. (Bowley, 2010). You're losing about 0.5 percent of your muscle mass a year (Kalman, 1990). To reverse these processes and stretch peak performance, your workouts now emphasize flexibility and power, without neglecting the aerobic component for cardio-vascular performance. In your 40s you may want to find interest in a yoga class once a week, a great way to concentrate on your muscles and posture, meditate, breath and releasing of tension. Studies show that practicing yoga can improve flexibility, relieve back pain, and reduce stress. Boston University researchers report that people who did yoga weekly boosted levels of the brain chemical GABA by 27 percent. Low levels of GABA have been linked to anxiety (Streeter, 2010). Practicing yoga can also help your body maintain its antioxidant levels, Indian researchers report (Sinha, 2007).

Exercises for the 40-50 year old man
Bending to sides

Starting position: Stand with legs more than shoulder-width apart, knees slightly bent, hold a band stretched over your head.

Bend your upper body deeply and slowly to the side, keeping your abs tucked in and your knees slightly bent. Go back to starting position.

How many? 10 to your right, 10 to your left, twice in a row.

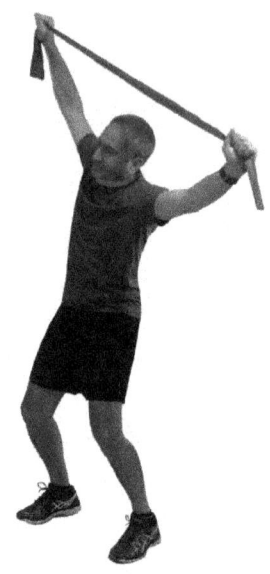

Stretching your chest

Starting position: stand with legs more than shoulder-width apart, knees slightly bent, place your hands together behind your back.

Bend your body forward and lift your arms up. Hold still that stretch for 10 sec and breathe regularly.

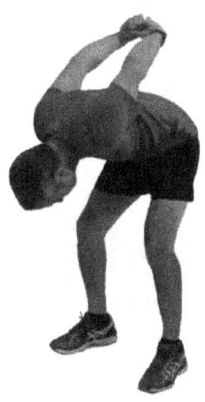

A hurdle stretch

Starting position: Sit in a hurdle position as shown – right thigh bent to your front and left thigh bent to your back.

Lean back with your body and feel a strong stretch on rear thigh. Hold position for 10 sec. and switch to the other leg.

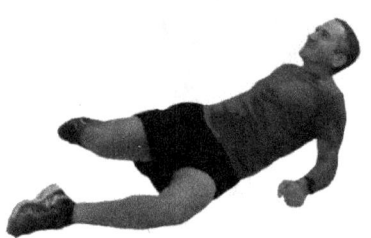

The Wells and Dillon (1952) "sit and reach" flexibility test

The "sit and reach" test is a common measure of flexibility and mainly measures the flexibility of the lower back and hamstring muscles. This test is important as because tightness in this area is implicated in lumbar lordosis, forward pelvic tilt, and lower back pain. First described by Wells and Dillon, (1952), it is now widely used as a general test of flexibility.

Remove your shoes and sit on a flat surface, legs extended in front of the body, toes pointing up and feet slightly apart, with the soles of the feet against the base of the step. (If there is no step, any flat surface will do). Place the ruler on the ground between your legs or on the top of the step. Place one hand on top of the other, and then reach slowly forward. At the point of your greatest reach, hold for a couple of seconds, and measure how far you have reached. If you have trouble straightening your legs, get a friend to help by holding the knees down flush with the ground. See also video demonstrations of the mark or take note of your best score, take a measurement in cm. or inches beyond the base of your foot, or if you did not reach your toes, measure how far before the feet you were (a negative measurement score).

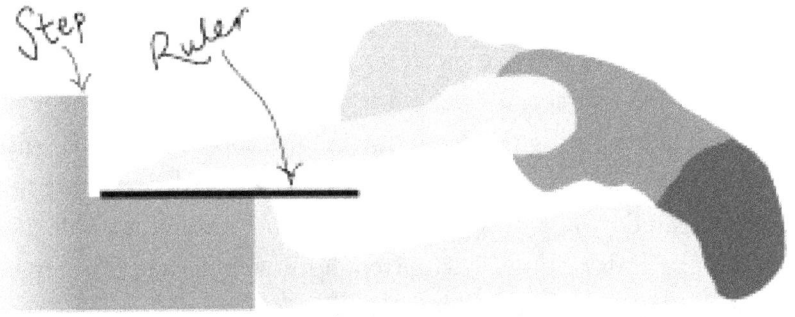

(Picture source: @topendsports.com)

Compare your results to the table:

	cm
super	> +27
excellent	+17 to +27
good	+6 to +16
average	0 to +5
fair	-8 to -1
poor	-20 to -9
very	< -20

Stretching is important at any given time during the day, not only after working-out. A study from Health Services, Merck, Wilson, NC suggests that continued development and implementation of stretching programs in the workplace may benefit employees by increasing flexibility and potentially preventing injuries due to muscle strains. Stretching programs in the workplace also may improve components of employees' perceptions of their physical bodies (Moore, 1998). Hence, the best time to stretch would be whenever your feel like it during the day. Stretching at your desk may be one simple way to keep moving, even as you stay seated. Sedentary time is best mitigated by lots of frequent movements, even if it's only done for brief periods of time. The current approach deriving from recent studies is that muscle stretching, whether conducted before, after, or before and after exercise, does not produce clinically important reductions in delayed-onset muscle soreness in healthy adults. (Herbert, 2011). However, as far as physical training is concerned, it is recommended to stretch after a work-out or at least when your muscles are warm (Bloch, 1998), (Woods, 2007).

Listen to your body. If you feel a good stretch is needed after a vigorous work-out - you stretch. Stretching after a workout is the most productive and safest time because the muscles are warm and pliable (Vindum, 2009).

It is highly recommended to warm up for at least 5 to 10 minutes before stretching.

Hold a stretch for 10 seconds, release for 5 seconds, and then execute the stretch again.

Inhale to prepare for a stretch, and exhale slowly while lengthening the muscle.

Stretching your hips

Starting position: Stand with legs more than shoulder-width apart, knees slightly bent, left hand on your hip and right hand straitened toward the ceiling.

Extend and reach the right arm up as you keep your abs tucked-in and bend your body to your left. Stay in position for 10 seconds and go back to starting position.

How many? 3 times in a row for each side.

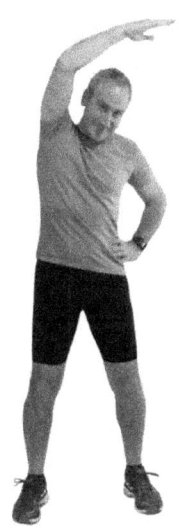

The Cat posture

Starting position: Stand with legs more than shoulder-width apart, knees slightly bent and place your hands on your thighs.

Perform a full curve of your back, keeping your chin close to your chest. Stay in position for 10 seconds and go back to starting position.

How many? 4 times in a row.

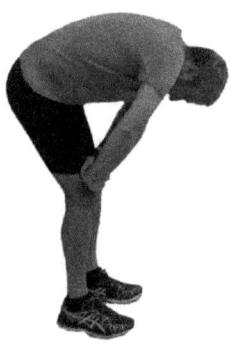

Walk on the spot

Starting position: get down to a push-up position, place your glutes high as shown.

Bring right ankle to the floor and when you feel a full stretch in your gastrocnemius - stay in position for 10 sec.

How many? Twice in a row for each side.

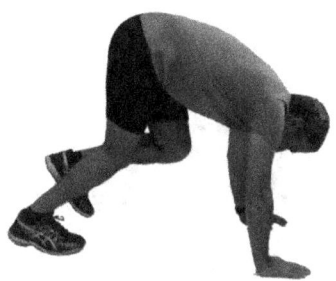

The child position

Starting position: Get down on your knees and place glutes on your ankles. Bend your body forward and place your arms down in front of you as shown. Your forehead should touch the floor.

How many? Stay in position for one minute.

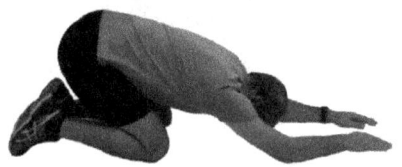

Put your strength to the test: How strong is your upper body?

In your 40s, strength in your upper body decreases by 60 percent in comparison to your previous decade (Runnels, 2005). It's important to strengthen your upper body in order to ease stress from the shoulder bend, to maintain posture and balance, to help perform everyday movements, and to prevent injuries. A simple way to determine how strong you are would be the push-up ultimate test:

Age	40-49
Excellent	34
Good	28-34
Above average	21-28
Average	11-20
Below average	6-10
Poor	1-5

That's the way to prove your score:

Find the number of repetitions you can perform in a row.

Divide that number in two. For instance if your score is 10, 5 is the number to perform in one set.

Perform 4 times per week 3 sets of 5 repetitions with a one minute break between sets.

Every week for 6 weeks take 10 seconds off of your break time till you are capable of preforming all 3 sets one after the other with zero breaks.

You are a woman in your 40s, the kids are older now and you can allow yourself to take care of you for a change. Metabolic rate declines significantly, and a potential gain of weight occurs if you don't watch your calorie intake (Toth, 1999). Perimenopause can begin in some women in their 30s, but most often it starts in women ages 40 - 44. It is marked by changes in menstrual flow and in the length of the cycle. The decline in estrogen after menopause can increase the risk for a number of health problems for women (heart disease, osteoporosis, mood changes, cognitive functions and memory loss, skin changes). A regular fitness program in your 40s underlines three components: joints flexibility, maintaining and increasing muscles mass and improving cardio-vascular abilities, so important for your heart's functions your mood and your balanced weight (Davis, 2008).

Exercises for the 40-50 year old woman
A band on your arms and abs.

Starting position: Stand with legs more than shoulder-width apart, knees slightly bent, place band behind your back holding it on both sides. Stretch the band forward and lift your knee at the same time towards your chest.

How many? 20 repetitions one knee after the other.

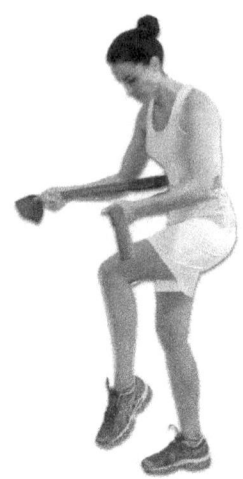

Strengthen your back and stretch your inner thighs.

Starting position: Sit with your legs wide spread and raise your arms up.

Bend your back forward and hold in position for 10 seconds.

Lean forward to release tension in your back and stay in position for 10 seconds.

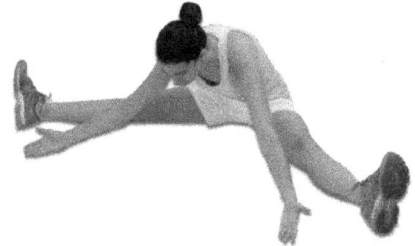

Stretch with a roll.

Starting position: Lie down on your back and place a roll horizontally along your lower back, as shown.

Gently and slowly roll back and forth on the roll for 30 seconds.

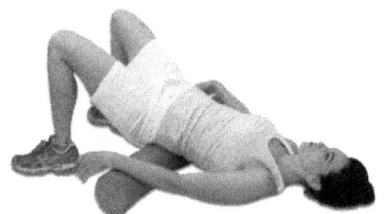

50s + : Balance, Coordination and Cardio

You are a 50 + year old man, at the prime of your life. Exercising regularly is your strongest medicine. In fact, according to a recent commentary in the Archives of Internal Medicine, physical activity may be the most effective prescription physicians can dispense for the purposes of promoting successful aging (Herring, 2010).

It's never too late to begin. A fascinating Swedish study examined how a change in level of physical activity after middle age influenced mortality and compared it with the effect of smoking cessation. Results were clear: Increased physical activity in middle age is eventually followed by a reduction in mortality to the same level as seen among men with constantly high physical activity. (This reduction is comparable with that associated with smoking cessation) (Byberg, 2009).

Exercise protects your heart, relaxes your arteries, makes your erections harder, builds muscle, strengthens your bones, fights cancer, boosts your immune system, and perhaps most inspiring, it's one of the best ways to rewire your brain. One of the unfortunate characteristics of the brain is that it generally shrinks and atrophies with advancing age. In fact, both the prefrontal cortex and hippocampus shrink at roughly 1% to 2% annually in individuals over the age of 55 (Raz, 2005). If you don't exercise, it's like your brain is in a cast, and your brain cells and networks atrophy (Ratey, 2008). Adults who devoted 4 days a week to an hour of moderate aerobic exercise, (running, stair climbing, or riding a stationary bike) had more blood flow in their dentate gyrus, the area of the brain where memories are formed, according to a Columbia University study. (Sahai, 2007). Increased blood flow may signal the growth of new brain cells, a process known as neurogenesis. It's also possible (Brickman, 2007) that exercise stimulates the release of a growth factor in the brain tied to neurogenesis. Another study found that people who did resistance training once a week saw a 12.6 percent jump in a performance on memory tests (Liu-Ambrose, 2010). Findings from a prospective study (Kwok, 2011) demonstrated how low-intensity level mind-body exercise, coordination exercise could be beneficial to the cognitive functioning and physical mobility of older adults.

After 50, the sedentary man's muscle loss speeds up, and he then loses about 10 percent of his muscle mass every decade. This leads directly to osteoporosis. If you've been lifting weights, keep it up. If you haven't, start now—it's not too late. Your workout should also involve more balance moves to strengthen your feet, ankles, and core and to straighten your posture.

Exercises for the 50+ year old man

1. Balance on 6.

Starting position: Down to a "Six-legged" position, arms shoulder-width apart.

Lift one arm forward and the opposite leg backward, as shown.

How many? Stay in position for one minute on each side.

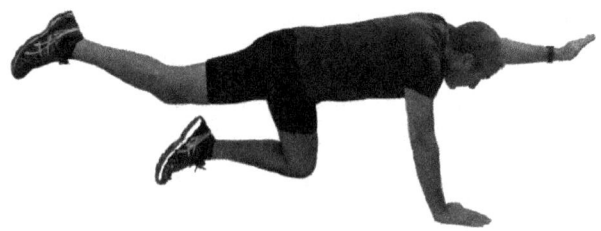

2. Straight bend for strength and stretch.

Starting position: Stand with legs more than shoulder-width apart, knees slightly bent, arms in a V position above your head, as shown.

Bring your upper body forward up to 45 degrees. as you keep your back unbent. Stay in position for 2 seconds and go back to starting position.

How many? 10 repetitions, 3 sets, a 30 sec. break between sets.

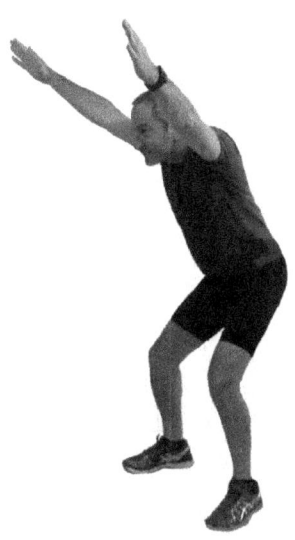

You are a 50 + year old woman, at the prime of your life. Physical activity is critical for your vitality, energy levels and over-all health. The average age that women reach menopause is 51 years, although it can occur as early as age 40 to as late as the early 60s. Women now have a life expectancy of more than 80 years (Matters, 2002). Currently, women can expect to live some 30 or 40 years of their life in the postmenopausal state. Menopause is not a disease. However, many conditions are associated with estrogen depletion, including heart disease, osteoporosis, and other complications. (Robin, 2013). Fortunately, effective treatments are available for these conditions. For protection against all aging diseases, you should pursue a lifestyle that includes a balanced aerobic and weight resistance exercise program appropriate to your age and medical conditions (Perrig-Chiello, 1998).

Brisk walking, stair climbing, hiking, dancing, and tai chi are all helpful. Several studies report that exercise can help control hot flashes (Pines, 2007). Evidence is also accumulating that coordinative exercises have profound benefits for brain function, including improvements in learning and memory as well as in preventing and delaying loss of cognitive function (Praag, 2009). A healthy diet plus regular, consistent exercise can also help ward off the weight gain associated with menopause. Weight-bearing exercises are specifically helpful for protecting against bone loss as well as maintaining and improving cognitive abilities (Rogers,1993), (Ferrari, 2013).

Exercises for the 50+ year old woman
Opening an energetic cycle.

Lie down on your back, open your knees and put your feet close together, as shown. Take three deep breathes, letting your knees open even wider and feel the inner thigh stretching. Stay in position for one minute.

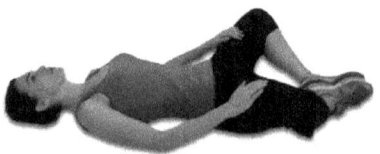

Balance and coordination.

Stand on your left foot, lift your right knee and your right arm. Extend your left arm to your left, as shown. Stay in position for 30 seconds and switch sides.

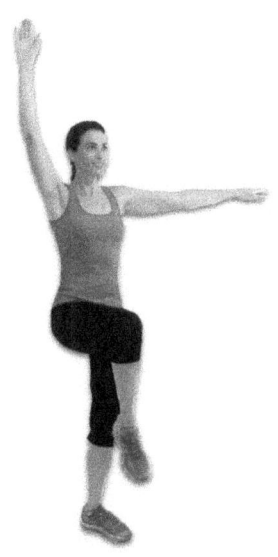

Your weekly training plan, (for men and women, 3 times a week):

Complete this 50-minute workout 3 days a week, and do the flexibility training every day.

5 minutes: warm up and preparing for action.	15 minutes: Power training	20 minutes: aerobic training	10 minutes: stretching and relaxation
5 min. warm-up of fast walk.	Resistance training should include all muscle groups.	Your goal is to burn fat and maintain your over-all health. You can perform a 20 minutes aerobic training (swimming, bike riding or walking) at an effort of 70 percent of your maximal pulse. A circuit or an interval training is recommended when you wish to improve your cardio-vascular abilities.	Make sure you stretch every muscle you have worked on during your work-out.

Make clockwise circles with your arms, starting with a small range of motion and working up to circles that use your full range of motion. Do 10 to 15 reps, and then reverse direction 10 torso rotations, swing tour arms from side to side. 10 hip circles for each direction. Take a deep breath three times.	You can use bands, fit-ball, TRX training and weights, as long as you keep it on a relatively high amount of repetitions on moderate resistance such as 50-60 % of your RM1. You do not want to overload and you simply wand to improve your muscle's strength.		Stay still in stretching position for at least 10 seconds and breathe all the way through your stretch.
	You can use machines on your local gym, attend a power class in a studio nearby, or embrace your own sets of exercises at home.		

Find your Balance

The loss of ability to balance may be linked with a higher risk of falling, increased dependency, illness, and sometimes early death (Wiley, 2011). Lack of exercise causes a loss of nerve sensitivity and loss of muscle strength. As you age, your balancing skills become less dependable, especially if you don't use them regularly. Staying physically active helps you keep your balance as you age. Evidence show that strength and balance training is safe and effective at reducing falls and improving lower extremity strength and balance in adults aged 50 years and older at high risk for falls, including patients with diabetic peripheral neuropathy (Tofthagen, 2012).

Are you doing enough to stay steady on your feet? Oprah Winfrey, (at Oprah.com), invites you to find-out how much your balance skills are affecting your functional age, by taking this simple static balance test.

Test: How long can you stand on one leg with your eyes closed before falling over?

1. Find a partner and a watch. Enlist the help of a friend or family member who has a watch with a second hand and five minutes to spare.

2. Take off your shoes. Stand barefoot on a flat, hard surface. Ask your partner to hold the watch and stand close by in case you start to fall.

3. Close your eyes. Lift one foot (left foot if right-handed, right foot if left-handed) about 6 inches off the floor, bending your knee at a 45-degree angle.

4. Lift your foot. Ask your partner to start timing.

5. Hold this position. Keep still as long as you can without jiggling or teetering, falling, or opening your eyes.

6. Stop the clock. Stop timing when the raised foot begins to lower or touch the ground, if you begin to sway or if you open your eyes.

7. Repeat the test three times. Note the number of each test and calculate the average of the three results.

8. Match the average to the chart below.

Static Balance Test: Results Chart	
Average Time	Equivalent RealAge
4 seconds	70
5 seconds	65
7 seconds	60
8 seconds	55
9 seconds	50
12 seconds	45
16 seconds	40
22 seconds	30-35
28 seconds	25-30

Improve your balance

Almost any activity that keeps you on your feet and moving will help preserve your body's balancing system. In particular, exercises that force your muscles to bear weight and overcome resistance will help support your joints and improve your stability.

Tai Chi, a gentle form of Chinese martial arts, focuses on slow sequential movements, providing a smooth, continuous and low intensity activity. It has been promoted to improve balance, strength, flexibility cardiorespiratory fitness, endurance and to reduce falls in the elderly, especially those at risk (Thornton, 2004).

Consult your doctor before beginning an exercise program for the first time, or if you have a medical condition that affects your ability to exercise safely.

On the balance board.

Starting position: stand on the balance board with your feet slightly spread and find your balance. You can use a chair to support your

109

body until you stand still.

Raise your arms in round circles as if you exhale deeply.

How many? 5 circles to one direction and 5 to the other, twice in a row. You fell off in the middle? Restart all over again until you fully succeed in performing.

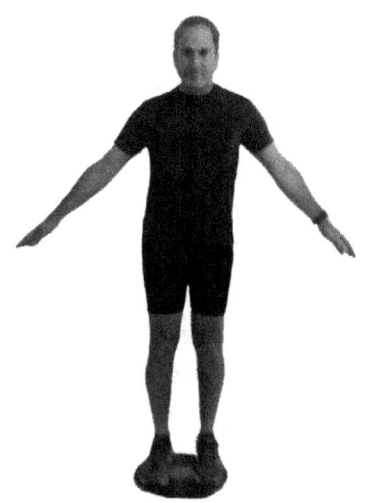

Classic balance

Starting position: Stand with legs more than shoulder-width apart, knees slightly bent.

Move your body weight to your right leg and lift your left leg straight back. Spread your arms to your sides, as shown. Stay in position for 5 seconds. .

How many? 5 seconds on each leg, twice in a row. Is it too easy for you? Stay for 10 seconds or more.

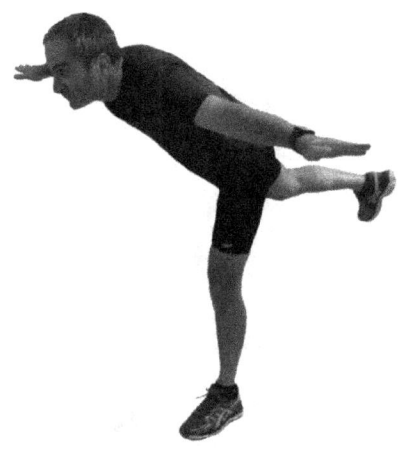

Sided Balance.

Starting position: Stand with legs more than shoulder-width apart, knees slightly bent. Raise both your arms up to a V shape. Maintain loose shoulders and remember to breathe.

Move your body weight to your right leg and lift your left leg to the side, 45 degrees off of the ground.

Stay in position for 5 seconds.

How many? 5 seconds for each leg, twice in a row. Is it too easy for you? Stay for 10 seconds or more.

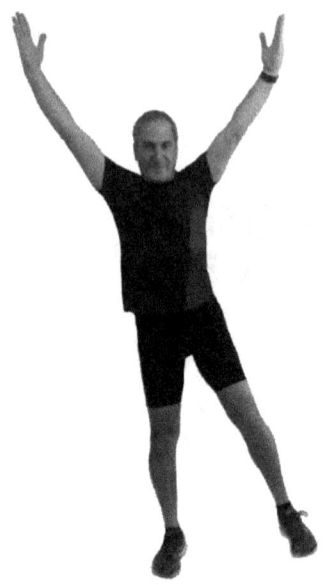

Static on the Bossu.

Starting position: Place one leg on the Bossu and lift the knee of the other leg toward your chest. Spread your arms to the sides to help maintain balance.

How many? Stay in position for as long as you can and write down your score. Perform with the other leg and compare the results of both sides.

Perform each side 3 times in a row and try to improve score of both sides.

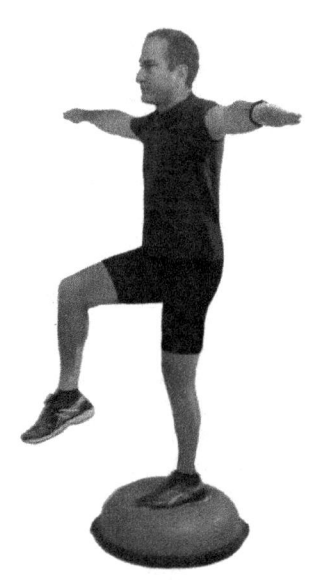

The power of Visualization and mental imagery: Work-in and work-out

Over the past 30 years or so, work in cognitive psychology, artificial intelligence and cognitive neuroscience have greatly advanced our knowledge of imagery. This is potentially very relevant to the problem of consciousness (Nigel, 1998). The concept of consciousness appears to have had little currency before the 17th century. Not only did philosophers before Rene Descartes fail to worry about how consciousness fitted into the natural world, they did not even claim to be conscious. If we are conscious, however, we must assume that they were, too, and it hardly seems plausible that they could have been unaware of it. When the mind was discussed in former ages, both before and within the work of Descartes and the study of consciousness, the concept of imagination filled most of the key conceptual roles that consciousness fills today, and continued to be used in these ways, long after the Cartesian revolution. (Descartes, 1996).

"Where the Mind goes, the body will follow" (Arnold Schwarzenegger)

Nowadays, almost everyone has heard of the mind-body connection. One of the key assumptions this book relate to is the belief that the words we use have a tremendous effect on our life and that even "spoken thoughts" may either "harm" or "heal". Austin's important work in "How to do things with words", (1962), as well as Perelman's new rhetoric based upon Aristotelian theory, defines "argumentation" as the ensemble of the spoken resources that the speaker uses in order to make an adhesion of an adversary to a certain thesis. (Declercq, 1992). Plantin, (1997), adds that "rhetoric is a discourse technique whose objective is to form an action: make somebody think, speak, be convinced or react".

Let's dig even deeper, beyond the words: Everywhere our mind goes, the body must follow. It's not a choice. Through a flood of chemical messengers, every thought we have is sent to our body. Therefore, our mind plays the major role in our goals, achievements, weight, aging, and life. (Chopra, 2009). Over the past two decades, much work has been carried out on the use of mental practice through motor imagery for optimizing the retraining of motor function in people with physical disabilities (Malouin, 2010). Mental imagery is defined as the use of the senses to recreate a physical experience in the mind (Dai, 2001). It's been shown to deliver some impressive results: during mental imagery, the electrical activity in the muscle we are thinking about is comparable to that measured during the actual movement itself (Lebon, 2008). And brain mapping studies (Reiser, 2011) show that similar parts of the brain are activated during both real and imagined movements.

The results from a study held at the University of Iowa add to existing evidence for the neural origin of increases in strength that occur before muscle hypertrophy. Strength increase was very clearly achieved without repeated activation of muscle (Yue, 1992). Another study, more recent and quite widely cited among researchers (Reiser,

2011), aimed to determine the magnitude of strength gains following high-intensity resistance training that can be achieved by imagery of the respective muscle contraction imagined maximal isometric contraction. It is concluded that high-intensity strength training sessions can be partly replaced by imagined maximal isometric contraction training sessions without any considerable reduction of strength gains.

In a study from the Department of Biomedical Engineering in Cleveland, subjects were able to make their arms stronger simply by imagining themselves doing curls. After 12 weeks of mental training (15 minutes per day, 5 days per week), strength in the imagery group had increased by 13.5%, which was significantly larger than the progress made by the control group. (Ranganathan, 2004).

The term "imagery" is slightly misleading, as we need to do more than just paint a mental picture. The most effective imagery involves duplicating the sights, sounds, feelings, thoughts, and emotions that we would experience during the actual event. We will deal with that technique in detail in chapter 3 as far as working on mental issues other than fitness. For now, we think of it as a mental movie that engages all of our senses: What can you hear? What can you smell? What do you see? It must be as real and vivid as you can make it.

"I also used a lot of visualization in biceps training. In my mind I saw my biceps as mountains, enormously huge, and I pictured myself lifting tremendous amounts of weight with these superhuman masses of muscle." (Schwarzenegger, 2012).

In a study from the Centre of Research and Innovation in Sport in Lyon, France (Lebon, 2010), subjects trained as usual, but spent the time between each set visualizing the exercise and imagining how the muscles would feel during each rep. The control group carried out a neutral task. The exact instructions given to the subjects were:

Imagine yourself performing the exercise with your eyes closed, by perceiving the different movements just as if you had a camera on your head, and feel the body's sensations. You have to see and feel only what you would see and feel if you had to perform this particular exercise. Imagine the movement using the most comfortable way for you, and make sure not to contract your muscles.

After 12 workouts, the mental imagery group had gained strength more quickly than the control group in one of the two exercises tested. They could do more reps with a given weight and lift more weight for a single repetition.

Mind Games at the GYM

Words have the power to change, create, and motivate not only "others" but also the self. In the study of narration and narrative levels, for instance, there is no such thing as a "monologue" since the speaker by definition communicates with himself (Rimmon-Kenan, 1983). Hence, there is always an interlocutor, an addressee, someone who is affected. You can talk to yourself and lift your own spirits. Mental imagery could also improve your performance simply by making you more confident that you can lift a certain weight.

Some additional mental strategies can help your mind push your body far beyond what you may believe you're capable of (Nilsson 2012):

Rewards: When it's starting to hurt and you are ready to quit, imagine you are offered a million dollars to do one more repetition.

Lighter weights: imagine the weight is less than it actually is. Imagine you are lifting a softball or a feather.

Magnetic force: If you're doing dumbbell presses, imagine they are two powerful magnets that are irresistibly drawn to each other. If you're curling, imagine your eyes as magnets attracting the bar towards them.

Pain management: To fight pain, tell yourself that it is not your pain -

it's somebody else's.

Self-Praise: Tell yourself how big and strong and powerful you are and how this weight is child's play.

Program that little voice in your head: Most people have a little voice in their head that warns them not to do things that may seem unreasonable or threatening, such as: You better not do that or you'll hurt yourself. You can't lift that much, let's quit. Reprogram that little voice to tell you things like: That felt pretty good, let's add more weight or You can do another rep. You can usually do more than you think you can, and you never know until you try. Don't automatically assume you'll never accomplish anything or you never will.

Competitions: Have competitions with a training partner or with yourself. Challenge yourself to break personal bests and reward yourself when you do. This type of competition can dramatically increase intensity.

Explosive imagery: Just before a set, put images of explosive power in your head, such as: Rockets, artillery, a stampede, explosions, etc. This form of imagery will start up your adrenaline and give you a little extra kick to get your set going. Imagine this explosive power rocketing the weights you are using.

Mind in muscle: Try to put your mind in the muscle you're working. Try to consciously fire the muscle fibers.

Donald Duck: If you find your inner voice speaking negatively, change the voice so it sounds like Daffy or Donald Duck. You won't be inclined to take it so seriously.

Mentor: Imagine you have a mentor or someone you are trying to impress standing over you and watching as you do your set. Imagine they are encouraging you and pushing you harder and harder.

Relaxation: not only after an intense work-out

Most people (watch them at the gym, or track your spouse arriving home after a good run, or just look in the mirror) are so pleased their training session is over, they hit the shower and continue on with their life. If they bother to stretch at the end of their work-out, it's a huge plus. Indeed, exercise of sufficient intensity and duration has been demonstrated to increase circulating beta-endorphins that serve as natural pain-killers and have positive psychological effects (Goldfarb, 1997), but relaxing your mind, (and really relaxing your muscles) after training your body is a Must. Not only did your body work in an exhausting and tiring way, but you also continue right on to your exhausting day or rest-of-the evening. Our fast-paced society can cause people to push their minds and bodies to the limit, often at the expense of physical and mental well-being. According to the Mind/Body Medical Institute at Harvard University, 60 - 90% of all medical office visits in the United States are for stress-related disorders (Arias, 2006). Such stress has damaging effects on health and the immune system. Relaxation techniques are helpful tools for coping with stress and promoting long-term health, in a different way than exercise, by slowing down the body and quieting the mind. Brief training in mindfulness meditation or somatic relaxation reduces distress and improves positive mood states (Jain, 2007).

Results from the 2007 National Health Interview Survey found that approximately one in nine children (11.8%) had used complementary and alternative medicine therapy over the past 12 months, with the most commonly used therapies being non-vitamin, non-mineral, natural products (3.9%) and chiropractic or osteopathic manipulation (2.8%). Children whose parent used complementary and alternative medicine were almost five times as likely (23.9%) to use complementary and alternative medicine as children whose parent did not use complementary and alternative medicine (5.1%). For both adults and children in 2007, when worry about cost delayed receipt of conventional care, individuals were more likely to use complementary and alternative medicine than when the cost of conventional care was not a worry. Between 2002 and 2007, increased use was seen among adults for acupuncture, deep breathing exercises, massage therapy, meditation, naturopathy, and yoga (Barnes, 2008). Used daily, these practices can lead to a healthier perspective on stressful circumstances. In fact, more than 3,000 studies show the beneficial effects of relaxation on health and well-being (Eppley, 1989), (Cahn, 2006).

Progressive relaxation: For this relaxation method, you focus on tightening and relaxing each muscle group: (Golombek, 2001).

Lay on your back, close your eyes. Feel your feet. Sense their weight. Consciously relax them and sink into the bed. Start with your toes and progress to your ankles.

Feel your knees. Sense their weight. Consciously relax them and feel them sink into the bed.

Feel your thighs. Feel their weight. Consciously relax them and feel them sink into the bed.

Feel your abdomen and chest. Sense your breathing. Consciously ask them to relax. Deepen your breathing slightly and feel your abdomen and chest sink into the bed.

Feel your buttocks. Sense their weight. Consciously relax them and feel them sink into the bed.

Feel your hands. Sense their weight. Consciously relax them and feel them sink into the bed.

Feel your upper arms. Sense their weight. Consciously relax them and feel them sink into the bed.

Feel your shoulders. Sense their weight. Consciously relax them and feel them sink into the bed.

Feel your neck. Sense its weight. Consciously relax it and feel it sink into the bed.

Feel your head. Sense its weight. Consciously relax it and feel it sink into the bed.

Feel your mouth and jaw. Consciously relax them. Pay particular attention to your jaw muscles and unclench them if you need to. Feel your mouth and jaw relax and sink into the bed.

Feel your eyes. Sense if there is tension in your eyes. Sense if you are forcibly closing your eyelids. Consciously relax your eyelids and feel the tension slide off the eyes.

Feel your face and cheeks. Consciously relax them and feel the tension slides off into the bed.

Mentally scan your body. If you find any place that is still tense, then consciously relax that place and let it sink into the bed (UMMC, 2011).

When we become stressed our bodies engage in something called the "fight or flight response": increased heart rate, blood pressure and rate of breathing, and a 300 - 400% increase in the amount of blood being pumped to the muscles (very similar to metabolic behavior due to work-out). Over time, these reactions raise cholesterol levels, disturb intestinal activities, and depress the immune system. In general, they leave us feeling "stressed out" (University of Maryland Medical Center, 2013). However, we also possess the opposite of the "fight or flight" response: the "relaxation response." This term, first coined in the mid-1970s by a Harvard cardiologist named Herbert Benson, refers to changes that occur in the body when it is in a deep state of relaxation (Benson, 1975). A study from the Division of Endocrinology and Molecular Medicine in Kentucky showed how the regular practice of Transcendental Meditation may have the potential to reduce systolic and diastolic blood pressure by approximately 4.7 and 3.2 mm Hg, respectively. These are clinically meaningful changes

(Anderson, 2008). These changes that occur in the body include decreased blood pressure, heart rate, muscle tension, and rate of breathing, as well as feelings of being calm and in control.

Al was suffering from anxieties and phobias. She came to my studio 5 years ago in order to lose some weight and get stronger in body and soul. She had been treated with Cipralex (used to treat depression, obsessive-compulsive disorder, (OCD), and generalized anxiety disorder, (GAD), prior to our Gymind process. Apparently Cipralex was not enough. Al understood the importance of exercise in her everyday life, in order to take control over her body and to feel stronger inside and out. The first time we went out of the studio for a good run was a WOW moment for both Al and me. A few minutes into the run, she stopped, petrified, and said: "This is exactly how I feel when I experience an anxiety attack: My pulse rate is high, I sweat, breathe fast ..." I reassured Al it was ok to keep on with our jogging session and promised that at the end of this cardio routine and long after we have finished, she would feel calm, in control, and peaceful.

Learning the relaxation techniques helps to counter ill effects of the "fight or flight" response and, over time, allows the development of a greater state of alertness. It is now a recommended treatment for many stress-related disorders. So, practicing relaxation techniques can reduce stress symptoms by: slowing heart rate; lowering blood pressure; slowing your breathing rate; increasing blood flow to major muscles; reducing muscle tension and chronic pain; improving concentration; reducing anger and frustration; boosting confidence to handle problems. (Mayo Clinic Stuff, 2011).

Relaxation is about breathing right, it's about getting enough sleep at night, and it's also a conscious state. Whatever makes you forget about your stress may relax you: a good movie, a long relaxing swim or a new recommended book you read. In the East, relaxation is attained by a number of practical techniques: Yoga, T'ai Chi, and

Meditation. So relaxation is a sort of physical training; you can also relax through movement.

While you move:

Concentrate on your breathing. Feel the oxygen entering deep into your cells, all over.

Imagine you are on soft ground, like walking on cotton or a cloud.

Soft music or the calming voice of your trainer can have a relaxing effect.

Think about the muscles that are engaged in your movement. Can you put less pressure there?

When you are done, lie down placing one hand on your chest and the other hand on your belly. Take a slow, deep breath, sucking in as much air as you can. As you're doing this, your belly should push against your hand. Hold your breath and then slowly exhale.

How to relax in 60 seconds and under?

Stress and tensions too heavy to handle? Meditation of any sort acts as an antidote to stress and helps you retake control over your body and mind. It may only take a minute:

Calibrate your state. How really stressed are you, on a scale from 1 to 10? (1. You are out of ice-cream in the refrigerator; 10. There is a threat of war with a foreign country). When you are aware of the level of your stress now, as opposed to other severe cases of stress (personal or national) that you have successfully managed, it puts things in perspective and instantly eases stress.

Grab a toy. You may know those cool office toys. Squeeze toys you can stretch, shape, and squish while you are at work. A nice distraction for your mind, to focus on the physical (ball, your hands), rather than the mental.

Hug. Hug your kids, your spouse, or a good friend. Hugs can melt you down in an instant. Oxytocin levels spike in your brain, and are also greatly stimulated during sex, birth, and breast feeding. (Psychologytoday.com)

Turn around. Not only on the carousel at the park, but also at your desk. Turn around with your chair. Impulses from the vestibular apparatus (a group of equilibrium receptors in the inner ear), travel to appropriate brain areas. This eventually has a calming effect. (Body Guide ADAM.com, 2011).

Seize the moment. You cannot change stressful situations. They are all there. But you can change the way your react to them. Look around and find something to admire: a beautiful flower, a beautiful song on the radio.

Reactivate your muscles. Engage in some push-ups or jump rope for a minute. This will release endorphins in your brain and will make you feel much more relaxed and concentrated.

Go on an imaginary vacation. Close your eyes, take three deep breaths, and imagine your last wonderful vacation. Hear what you heard, feel what you felt, see what you saw. Feel the wind in your hair, try and remember the taste of that lobster you ate at dinner time. Make that picture brighter, more colorful, more powerful, and own it. Link your thumb and finger together and anchor that picture in your body. This physiological "anchoring" will serve you later on, each time you are stressed: Simply link your fingers together, and you are retaking your vacation.

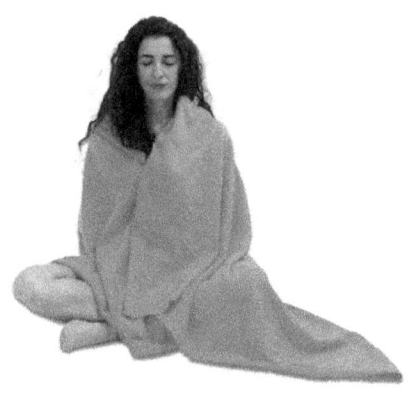

"You are retaking your vacation"

Turn upside down. Lie down on a fit-ball on your back so that you see the world upside down. This is a great way to stretch your pectoral muscles and your shoulders, but it also changes the perspective in your mind. For a minute you lose your sense of direction, you stretch, breathe, and calm down.

Eat chocolate. Cocoa and chocolate have been recognized as significant sources of phytochemicals with healthful effects. Go for dark chocolate over milk chocolate, aiming to get 70 % cocoa if possible. Chocolate contains phenethylamine (PEA), a molecule that resembles amphetamine and some other psychoactive stimulants. It contains small amounts of the amino acid tyramine that powerfully induces the release of adrenaline (Wenk, 2010). These foods are among the most concentrated sources of the procyanidin flavonoids, catechin and epicatechin. These flavonoids have potent antioxidant and antiplatelet effects following consumption of cocoa or chocolate (Keen, 2001).

Start to write. Start with all the bad things, just pour them all out, empty and release your mind of all the stressful things. When you are done, throw what you've just written into the garbage and start over. This time just focus on all the good things in your life and write them down. Concentrating on the nicer things makes them more meaningful and "magnetizes" good thoughts, hence good things, in your life. .

Did you remember to breathe today?

Stop for a second and wonder: Did you really breathe today? Have you taken a deep breath focusing on yourself, (or in yourself), rather than on the outside world? When you work-out, do you also work-in? Our hectic life-style, missions, "to-do's", meetings, chores – they are all part of this extended race through life. Unlike a jogging routine where you put on your running shoes, take control of your body, take charge and run, in the race of life we are only one part of this whole game, dependent on others. We are sometimes stressed out, sometimes even lost. We forget how much we need to inhale and exhale, release tensions accumulating in our body, so that we can recharge our batteries and continue. Stress and mental tension cause muscles to contract and have a bad influence on our immune system (Dusek and Benson, 2009).

Doesn't breathing come naturally for us? Why do we need to concentrate on an action so natural and intuitive?

It's just like with walking, running, or strength training, whether it's a natural movement or not: When you concentrate on the process, when your mind takes part of the action, you raise efficiency, improve effects, and maximize results (Lebon, 2008).

Engage in taking deep breath not only during, before, or after work-outs. A study from Columbia University College of Physicians and Surgeons in New York provides clinical evidence for the use of yoga breathing in the treatment of depression, anxiety, post-traumatic stress disorder, and for victims of mass disasters. By inducing stress resilience, breath work enables us to rapidly and compassionately relieve many forms of suffering (Brown, 2009). An Indian study shows that deep breathing exercise, even for a few minutes duration, is beneficial for the lung functions (Sivakumar, 2011).

Not yet the end: Know yourself, set a goal and choose a fitness plan that meets your needs

Going through this chapter we have met some people at a glance, enough to realize they are all very different from one another, yet they all are pursuing the same goal, (to be healthy), and they all utilize the same means, (physical training): 32-year-old Miller who loves to swim; Hana (22) who found comfort in her "20 minutes and you're done" routine; 45-year-old Aida who was once afraid of running due to old injuries; 12-year-old Tom who chose the pedometer as a great tool of motivation, along with Belle (27) and Leroy (29); Gabrielle who was compelled to walk for her health; Barak the acupuncturist whose training program enables him to regain control over his life; Dear 29-year-old Maya who embraces cardio-vascular activities as well as power training to repair her heart; Oliver the (former) hypotonic young boy, saved by exercising and strong will power; Liana's family who changed their attitude towards physical activity thanks to the needs of their obese 4-year-old; Muriel (22) who lost almost 40 kg. and "cannot skip a training session" as she was quoted in a health magazine; Irene (37), who fights Lupus by "being stronger" than the lupus is... Just like Nancy who knows she is allergic to soy products, even though "a billion Chinese cannot be wrong" and is pursuing the diet she feels is right for her. This chapter tells you to get in touch with your inner compass and get to know yourself, listen to your body, and follow your needs. Define your health, your goals, and enjoy the benefits of a "personalized work-out" (a la Agus's "personalized medicine"). Since nothing about working-out is "one size fits all", refer to this chapter as an inspirational methodology which calls you to take charge, set a goal, and choose a plan that fits you.

We are about to follow some of these people in the next two chapters. We will meet some more wonderful individuals, aspiring to see a whole picture about the body-mind connection and the holistic way to attain health.

Chapter II

Nutrition, Awareness and Body-Image

Primary thoughts and some proven facts: Eating smart for your health

People engage in eating behavior as a matter of survival every day. We have to make choices about what to eat, when, and how much. In contrast to our ancestors, whose primary task was to seek out any food that would provide energy and nutrients, those choices have become more difficult nowadays. In Western or westernized societies in particular, food is abundant, cheap, and available in a great variety (Meule, 2013). When we are energy-deficient, a complex interplay of physiological processes signals the brain that food should be consumed (we feel hungry). When enough food has been consumed, these processes signal that consumption should be terminated (we feel satiated or full). (Benelam, 2009). This regulation of eating is steadily challenged and overridden by the omnipresence of food and food-related cues. That is, eating can be triggered even in the absence of hunger or can be extended beyond satiation (Lowe, 2007). Numerous factors are known to determine or guide eating behavior in an automatic and implicit fashion (Cohen, 2008). Food choices and consumption are strongly influenced by environmental factors, such as advertising, packaging, portion sizes, also other people and sound, temperature, smell, color, time, lighting. (Stroebele, 2004). Constant monitoring and self-regulation of eating is necessary in order to eat healthily and to provide the body both qualitatively and quantitatively with the right nutrients. At the same time, eating healthily also means to be able to enjoy the rewarding aspects of food without falling prey to a loss of control over eating (Meule, 2013).

"An apple a day keeps the doctor away", a fact most kids are familiar with from a very young age. Now, as grown-ups, we are fully aware of the importance of eating good/feeling good/looking good. We may even be flooded with information: magazines, (Women's Health, Men's Health, Self, Fitness…), TV shows, (the former Oprah show, Tyra Banks show, Allan…), reality shows, (The Biggest Loser, Hell's Kitchen, Master Chef, Top Chef…), endless websites of recipes, nutritionists, success stories about weight-loss. They all represent this current era of awareness, knowledge and "media for the masses" as far as food, health and glamor are concerned. Nutrition plays such an important role in every part of our health, from disease to weight issues to life expectancy. And it's a proven fact. So we can't live on processed foods and factory-made foods and expect to have normal health (Fuhrman, 2003). A 12-year follow-up of a study from Boston found a significant positive association between the Western dietary pattern (higher intakes of red and processed meats, sweets and desserts, french fries and refined grains) and the risk of colon cancer (Fung, 2003) Our body uses food as fuel to operate at maximum efficiency. The better the fuel, the better our body runs. While it can survive on a diet of french-fries, soda, or processed meats, we pay a price (Agin, 2008).

Obesity occurs over time when we eat more calories than we use. A combination of dramatic change in eating habits and daily exercise results in weight loss, including a 60 percent reduction in the chance of developing chronic ailments, such as diabetes, heart disease, stroke, arthritis, and some cancers (Fuhrman, 2003), (Vastag, 2004). A high body mass index is associated with an increased risk of mortality from coronary heart disease (Dexter, 2013). The prevalence of clinically severe obesity is alarmingly increasing in the Western world. The widely published trends for overweight/obesity underestimate the consequences for physician practices, hospitals, and health plans because comorbidities and resulting service use are much higher among severely obese individuals. Accommodating severely obese patients will no longer be a rare event, and providers have to prepare to treat such patients on a regular basis (Sturm,

2003). A study conducted in Atlanta found that smoking is still the leading cause of mortality, but poor diet and physical inactivity may soon overtake tobacco as the leading cause of death. These findings, along with escalating health care costs and aging population, argue persuasively that the need to establish a more preventive orientation in the US health care and public health systems has become more urgent (Mokdad, 2004). Calorie restriction is the most effective and reproducible intervention for increasing lifespan (Hursting, 2003), which means that lean people live longer. (Manson, 1995). In the Nurses' Health Study, researchers examined the association between body mass index and overall mortality and mortality from specific causes in more than 100,000 women. Body weight and mortality from all causes were directly related among these middle-aged women. Lean women did not have excess mortality. The lowest mortality rate was observed among women who weighed at least 15 percent less than the U.S. average for women of similar age and among those whose weight had been stable since early adulthood. If you are obese, losing even 5 to 10 percent of your weight can delay or prevent some of these diseases. For example, that means losing 10 to 20 pounds if you weigh 200 pounds (Vastag, 2004).

Eating smart will help you get there. Foods contain combinations of nutrients and other healthful substances. No single food can supply all nutrients in the amounts you need. For example, oranges provide vitamin C but no vitamin B12; cheese provides vitamin B12 but no vitamin C. Eating large quantities of high-nutrient foods, according to Fuhrman (2003), is the secret to optimal health and permanent weight control: we must consume a high nutrient-per-calorie ratio. To make sure we get all of the nutrients and other substances needed for health, we have to choose the recommended number of daily servings from each of the five major food groups: grains, vegetables, fruits, milk, meat and beans.

More than that, according to Dr. Oz, (2012), a cardiovascular surgeon and "America's sweetheart" doctor, our body has a tremendous ability to heal through nutritional excellence, and unlike for many diseases, the cure for obesity is known.

Yet, the overabundance of diet books has created a complex and contradictory array of choices for those who are desperate to lose weight, for those who wish to eat smart. What to eat? How much? What is wrong? What is right? Proteins only? Whole grains only? No sugar? Gluten free? This chapter does not necessarily aim to explore every single diet plan that exists out there. We have enough of that, we are flooded with information. The chapter, representing the Gymind viewpoint, wishes to invite you to find your own path in that sea of nutritional endless opportunities through a full understanding of how important nutrition is for our health and identity, (you are what you eat), thanks to an intense and intelligent look at case-studies.

Skinny fat, a plausible oxymoron

"Could we schedule a session?" a thin, impressive 30-something-year-old woman approached me years ago. I gave her a surprised and flattering look, saying "What do you need ME for?" "I need to eat healthy, I need to exercise. I feel fat." Ili, that was her name, had a good solid BMI of 20 and something. She was really thin: 55 kg on a 1.65 height. Yet, when we checked her body fat percentage using an electronic caliper and a simple body-fat percentage scale, I was amazed to discover the number 32. Ili was thin, but according to her body fat percentage, she was fat.

The existence of a subgroup of normal-weight individuals displaying obesity-related phenotypic characteristics was first proposed in 1981. These individuals were identified as metabolically obese but of normal weight. It means they are under lean but over fat, not enough muscle and too much fat (especially belly fat, but not necessarily. With Ili it was spread all over her body). It was hypothesized that these individuals might be characterized by insulin resistance, high blood pressure, and higher cardiovascular risk despite having a body mass index (BMI) < 25 kg/m2. Studies found that the prevalence of the normal-weight individuals syndrome ranges between 5% and 45%, depending on the criteria used, age, BMI, and ethnicity. When compared with control subjects, they display an altered insulin sensitivity, a higher abdominal and visceral adiposity, higher blood pressure, and a lower physical activity energy expenditure. They are at higher risk for type 2 diabetes and cardiovascular diseases (Conus, 2007). A more recent study of 10 years follow-up from Korea talks about a higher mortality in metabolically obese normal-weight people than in metabolically healthy obese subjects (Choi, 2013). What once was the common wisdom that if you are overweight you are unhealthy, and if you are thin, you are healthy, is now known to be wrong. We now know how dangerous being skinny can be if you are a "skinny fat" person. While 68 percent of the American population is overweight, and most have diabetes (being somewhere on the continuum of pre-diabetes to Type 2 diabetes), it's now a proven fact, according to a study from the Department of Preventive Medicine, Northwestern University in Chicago, that nearly 1 in 4 skinny people have pre-diabetes and are "metabolically obese" (Carnethon, 2012). If you are a skinny fat person and are diagnosed with diabetes, your risk of death is double that of what it would be if you are overweight when diagnosed with diabetes.

The treatment for the skinny fat syndrome is the same as the cure for someone who is overweight with diabesity (obesity + diabetes). Gymind for Ili was, first and foremost, a process of eating healthy and strengthening her heart and body. Hyman (2012), suggests some practical moves:

Eat a low-glycemic load diet: Lean animal protein (chicken, fish, and eggs), nuts, seeds, beans, vegetables, fruits, and small amounts of non-gluten grains. (Brand-Miller, 2005).

Power up with protein: Start the day with protein and eat some at each meal. This makes your metabolism run hotter and cuts hunger.

Incorporate eggs, protein shakes, nuts, seeds, chicken, or fish.

Avoid the deadly white powder or flour: Including gluten-free flour products. Even whole grain flour acts like sugar in your body.

Beware of Frankenfood: Factory-made foods are often science projects with fake ingredients, including MSG (which causes ravenous hunger and is hidden as "natural flavoring"), high fructose corn syrup, artificial colors, preservatives, and chemicals.

Get the right oil: Eat omega-3 fat-rich foods, including sardines and wild salmon and avoid refined and processed vegetable oils except olive oil.

Get going and get strong: Both cardio and strength training are key. Cardio builds fitness and improves metabolism, and strength training builds muscle so you avoid becoming a skinny fat person (Umpierre, 2011).

Protect sleep time: Sleep deprivation alters metabolism and increases cravings for carbs and sugar. Sleep is sacred. Make your bedroom a sleeping temple and stay there for 7 to 8 hours a night.

Whether we are in the normal-weight group, the skinny-fat group or the over-weight group, we must fuel our body in the right way, relevant and adequate for us.

Going on a "diet", the smart way for you

"Being on a diet" does not necessarily mean "trying to lose weight". The etymology of the word "diet" derives from the ancient Greek δίαιτα (diaita) meaning "daily allowance, regulation, daily order". Yet we so frequently use this term for weight-loss purposes. We so often refer to calorie restrictions, fasting, diet pills, foods we don't love (since the ones we do love, doughnuts or fries, are out of the equation). We may develop a serious "resistance" to the word "diet", which is simply and nothing but a "daily allowance, regulation, daily order".

"I am so tired of dieting" said Emma, 55 years old. I have tried every single "diet on the menu" that life had to offer me. In a nutshell: pills, sprays, "color diet", cabbage soup diet, The Atkins Diet[3], detox... You name it. I have had enough. I love eating so much, what do I do? Am I doomed to stay fat and frustrated all my life"?

This is one of many monologues I have encountered over the years, since Emma only expresses what people feel and deal with in everyday life. Emma has not found the smart, adequate, suitable right path for her, yet. She was overwhelmed with too many "diet trends" up to a point that she almost gave up on good looks and good health. "Les régimes? C'est out !" (Diets? It's out!), says the Côté Santé French magazine (2012). They lead to frustration, to the "yoyo effect" (losing weight, then gaining it all back and losing again and so forth), and we have to avoid them. Find the right and adequate lifestyle for yourself, that's the way to go. Your "healthy weight" will follow.

Diet is not about willpower; it is about knowledge and conscious decisions

Knowledge is great power (Agus, 2012). We have already discussed in Chapter One the importance of knowing what's right for your body as far as exercising is concerned and listening to your body's needs. Your local city-hall library is overloaded with books, videos, and information dealing with working-out and fitness programs. But what is the right program for *you*? The same goes for foods and flavors, with dieting and recipes: what is good for *you*? Be a "wise consumer",

---

3 The Atkins diet, and other diets rich in animal products and low in fruits and unrefined carbohydrates, is likely to significantly increase a person's risk of colon cancer (Slattery, 1998). Scientific studies show a clear and strong relationship between cancers of the digestive tract, bladder and prostate with low fruit consumption (Bostick, 1994). What good is a diet that lowers your weight but also dramatically increases your chances of developing cancer? (Chen, 1998), (Fuhrman, 2003).

a "food critic", the closest friend of your palate, taste buds, stomach, and needs. This chapter invites you to be inspired by others, who are involved in that search, as we all are, for the right way to eat, in a world of endless opportunities and possibilities. The key to success is to know your needs and act accordingly.

It's never too late to decide and make a change in life. Remember that Swedish break-through research that found how "rehabilitated" 55-year-olds who, at a relatively late stage of life, chose to begin exercising to enjoy a healthy and long life at the same level as seen among men with constantly high physical activity (Byberg, 2009). Unlike Oliver the hypotonic kid, not all of us had the chance to begin from childhood. It does not mean we cannot begin now. By arming ourselves with solid knowledge and making changes to our current lifestyle, we have a fair chance to live longer. Surely we want to live a better quality of life (Agin, 2008).

It's not necessarily what you eat; it's when you eat

Matt, 48, pediatrician, married to a nurse, father of three, has been a client of mine since August 2008. His goal was to lose weight and get in shape: "I want to feel better about myself," he said, and those 94 kg (on 1.82 meters) don't help me do that". When I asked him about his eating habits, it turned out that at home his family maintains a very healthy kitchen, since two of his kids are "gluten-free" and the awareness of a healthy diet is always present. However, since he works very long hours at the clinic and manages a stressful schedule, Matt does not eat all day long. It's only at 20:00 or 21:00 and sometimes even later, that he eats a huge meal, compensating for a day of fasting.

"You are no less important than your patients," I said. "You may even become a better doctor the minute you start taking care of yourself, beginning with eating. You will have more patience, you will feel less stressful, and you will lose weight". Matt gave me a skeptical look, saying, "Does it matter if I eat 2000 calories in one meal or 6 meals during the day for a total of the same 2000?" I nodded, challenging him to try it just for one week. His wife was asked to prepare small meals to go, healthy snacks to carry along, and lots of water. The following week Matt wore a huge smile, after dropping 4 kilograms just by spreading out his calories and fueling his body throughout the day.

It has been well established that the circadian clock plays a crucial role in the regulation of almost every physiological process, including those of obesity and diabetes (Richards, 2013), so that disruption of circadian rhythms are correlated with obesity, brain dysfunctions, cardiovascular diseases, and metabolic disorders.(Mi Shi, 2012). Scientists at the Hebrew University of Jerusalem tested the effects of timing and fat intake on four groups of mice over an 18-week period to determine whether careful scheduling of meals could lower the effects of a high-fat diet. (Sherman, 2012). Notice that the research is actually on mice, and researchers were trying to determine if the body clock could have an impact on metabolism which, in turn, could affect factors such as body fat. The mice that had been fed a high-fat diet at regular intervals finished the trial in better condition than those that ate low-fat foods whenever they wanted, despite both groups consuming the same number of calories overall. The study confirms that improving metabolism through the careful scheduling of meals, without limiting the content of the daily menu, could be used as a therapeutic tool to prevent obesity in humans. (Froy, 2013). A promising interpretation of the results is that it may be possible to 'train' your metabolism. If you eat your three meals at the same time every day, your metabolism 'knows' to work harder to burn off the fat. This research has caught the attention of the media, but the findings do not mean that people should feel free to work a diet high in saturated fats, such as chips, curries, and burgers into every meal plan even if they are doing so at specific and regular times of the day. Eating at regular times may mitigate some of the health risks associated with a high-fat diet, but only to a very limited extent. Sadly for fans of high-fat fast food, it is very much *not* a case of 'It's not what you eat, it's when you eat'.

While sticking to mealtimes and not snacking between meals may be a good idea, it is preferable if meals contain a high proportion of fruit and vegetables and balanced amounts of carbohydrate and proteins that are low in sugar and saturated fats. High-fat diets and obesity are clearly linked to cardiovascular disease and many other chronic diseases and cannot be recommended. We assembled for Matt a potential nutrition plan that suited his life-style as a busy pediatrician, and "trained" his metabolism to use fats as an energy resource throughout the day:

A possible nutrition plan for Matt; ~ 1800 kcal.

Breakfast 7:00: Rushes out to work : an energy bar (120 kcal) and a yogurt (60 kcal), or two slices of whole wheat bread (80 kcal each) with cottage cheese (two spoons 60 kcal) or with avocado (half, 150 kcal) and a cup of coffee (with one tsp. of brown sugar 50 kcal). (Total of 250 kcal).

9:30, between patients: A banana and an apple (80, 60 kcal.), or a handful of walnuts (150 kcal), or a handful of almonds (150 kcal), or three dates. (150 kcal.).

11:30, between patients: A banana and an apple (80, 60 kcal.), or a handful of walnuts (150 kcal) or a handful of almonds (150 kcal), or three dates. (150 kcal.).

13:00, quick lunch, before a surgery at the hospital or a board meeting or continuing his day at the private clinic: Chicken breast in a whole wheat sandwich or 2 boiled eggs in a whole wheat sandwich or a Tuna whole wheat sandwich (250-400 kcal).

15:00, a quick coffee break: a cup of coffee and an energy bar (50, 120).

17:00, between patients: A banana and an apple (80, 60 kcal.) or a handful of walnuts (150 kcal) or a handful of almonds (150 kcal) or three dates. (150 kcal.).

19:00, dinner at home (see below) or between patients: a banana and an apple (80, 60 kcal.), or a handful of walnuts (150 kcal), or a handful of almonds (150 kcal), or three dates. (150 kcal.).

21:00, dinner at home: A bowl of brown rice (8 tbsp. 320 kcal), a vegetable salad (50 kcal), a grilled fish (100 kcal), or chicken breast (150 kcal).

If there were no nuts in any meal during the day, add two "Brazil nuts" and 7 "California nuts".

Is it OK to eat at night?

For Matt this question is irrelevant since his only chance of eating a warm homey meal is at night after a long hectic day as a successful pediatrician. Thanks to some minor yet crucial changes in his eating habits, combined with physical work-out throughout the week, he manages to keep his weight off so that he can enjoy a healthy life-style. However, recent studies explore how our natural metabolism is influenced by "Light at night".

In recent years we have shifted away from the naturally occurring solar light cycle in favor of artificial and sometimes irregular light schedules produced by electric lighting. Exposure to unnatural light cycles is increasingly associated with obesity and metabolic syndrome (Fonken, 2013), (Obayashi, 2013). A study from Spain supports the hypothesis that behavioral (sleep duration, eating patterns, and chronobiological characteristics) and hormonal (plasma ghrelin and leptin concentrations) factors explain the association between the Circadian Locomotor Output Cycles Kaput and weight loss. (Garaulet, 2011). This is highly related to the proven fact that reduced amounts of sleep are associated with overweight and obese status. Interventions manipulating total sleep time could elucidate a cause-and-effect relationship between insufficient sleep and obesity (Vorona, 2005), (Gangwisch, 2005), (Bixler, 2005).

Now we know that night eating syndrome, first identified in 1955 by Stunkard, a psychiatrist specializing in eating disorders (Cleator, 2012), is considered a dysfunction of circadian rhythm with a disassociation between eating and sleeping. If you eat regularly during the day and significantly increase your intake in the evening or nighttime, (if at least 25% of food intake is consumed after the evening meal, or at least two episodes of nocturnal eating per week), you are in that category of "night eating syndrome". An important recent addition to core criteria includes the presence of significant distress or impairment in functioning. This is a disturbing phenomenon that calls for further investigation as far as its relationship with traumatic life events, psychiatric comorbidity, the age of onset of Night Eating Syndrome, and the course of Night Eating Syndrome over time (Cleator, 2012). In the Medical Scientist Training Program in the University of Pennsylvania School of Medicine, Philadelphia, researchers found that in patients who had been treated for both Night Eating and headache by the same doctor, 29% were "not at all satisfied" with the treatment of their headache as compared to 76% who were "not at all satisfied" with their treatment of Night Eating. (Goncalves, 2009). This study does not necessarily refer to Night Eating Disorder as a mental disorder, but more as a behavioral element that should be identified when aiming for a healthy life-style and a normal weight.

Most of us start off the day with the best intentions for eating healthy. Unfortunately, a missed alarm, getting stuck in traffic, or working through the lunch hour can botch the best plans for eating right. With today's hectic schedules and an abundance of convenience foods, it's easy to get off track even when you want to stay on course. However, seizing eating at a certain hour can help you regain control over the situation.

Hanna, finding comfort in her "20 minutes and you're done" routine we have met in previous chapter; 45 years old Aida who once was afraid of running due to old injuries and many more could testify (yours truly included), how seizing to eat at a reasonable hour, 3-4 hours before bed-time, is the key to success as far as losing excessive weight and maintaining a healthy regime.

Hanna's nutrition plan; seizing to eat at 19:00 o'clock

Hanna is not highly physically active during the day; she assists her father the dentist in his clinic almost every day and is studying hard to get accepted to med school. She does work-out 20 minutes a day, fully aware of the importance of cardiovascular and strength training. Hanna is petite, 55 kg on 152 cm, and her goal was to reach a healthy fat percentage, maintain her body strength, and weight 45 kg. Hanna shared with me the fact that she had known "since forever" that eating at night really made it difficult for her to lose the weight and keep it off.

"I would go to bed feeling bloated and wake up in the morning angry at myself for eating at night, even if it was social eating in pleasant circumstances. I must put a stop to that, in addition to eating right during the day and working out".

This is an example of a potential nutrition plan, ~ 1200 kcal we fixed for Hanna:

8:00: 200 kcal: 2 Brazil nuts, 5 California nuts, 7 almonds and a handful of cranberries.

10:30: 160 kcal: Fiber 1 (1 cup) and 20 grams of 60 % cacao chocolate flakes.

13:30: 300 kcal: Brown rice (6 tbsp.), 1 low-fat corn schnitzel.

15:30: 200 kcal: 10 rice crackers with 5 % cheese (2 tsp.).

17:00: 60 kcal: an apple.

19:00 250 kcal: 1 boiled egg, a vegetable salad, and one boiled potato.

Fitness and Nutrition: Determine your goal, create your dish

For Matt, Hanna, Aida, and all the individuals we encountered in Chapter One as people who found comfort in exercising and physical activity, if their diet plan isn't what it needs to be, then achieving their goal to lose weight will fail completely. No matter how perfect their fitness activity, they will miss their health goal. Muriel, for example, (22, who lost almost 40 kg and embraced a sportive life-style), could be using the single greatest workout program ever created and it would get her absolutely nowhere if she did not eat in a way that supported her goals. The diet we eat accordingly is equally as important as our workout routine, if not more so, in terms of achieving our goal.

Find your Basal Metabolic Rate (BMR)

Our BMR is the amount of calories we'd burn if we stayed in bed all day (Agin, 2008). A critical step would be to learn about our BMR or RMR (resting metabolic rate) in order to recognize our own daily caloric needs so that we can balance eating and exercise accordingly. Once we know our BMR, we can calculate our daily calorie needs.

Calculations are different for men and women.

Men: BMR = 66 + (13.7 x weight in kilos) + (5 x height in cm) - (6.8 x age in years).

Women: BMR = 65 + (9.6 x weight in kilos) + (1.8 x height in cm) - (4.7 x age in years).

The Harris-Benedict Equation is a formula that uses our BMR and then applies an activity factor to determine our total daily energy expenditure (calories). In the early part of the 20th century, numerous studies of human basal metabolism were conducted at the Nutrition Laboratory of the Carnegie Institution of Washington in Boston, Mass, under the direction of Francis G. Benedict. Prediction equations for basal energy expenditure were developed from these studies. The expressed purpose of these equations was to establish normal standards to serve as a benchmark for comparison with basal energy expenditure of persons with various disease states, such as diabetes, thyroid, and other febrile diseases. The Harris-Benedict equations remain the most common method for calculating basal energy expenditure for clinical and research purposes (Frankenfield, 1998). The accuracy of this formula to predict dietary energy needs is affected by weight history status, according to a study published in Nutrition Research (Douglas 2007), suggesting that formulas used to calculate energy needs should take into account weight history and ethnicity.

If you are sedentary (little or no exercise) : Calorie-Calculation = BMR x 1.2

If you are lightly active (light exercise/sports 1-3 days/week) : Calorie-Calculation = BMR x 1.375

If you are moderately active (moderate exercise/sports 3-5 days/week) : Calorie-Calculation = BMR x 1.55

If you are very active (hard exercise/sports 6-7 days a week) : Calorie-Calculation = BMR x 1.725

If you are extra active (very hard exercise/sports & physical job or 2x training) : Calorie-Calculation = BMR x 1.9

Total Calorie Needs: Example:

If you are sedentary, multiply your BMR (1745) by 1.2 = 2094. This is the total number of calories you need in order to maintain your current weight.

Once we know the number of calories needed to maintain our weight, we can easily calculate the number of calories we need to eat in order to gain or lose weight. Eating should be enjoyable, but it should also serve to keep us looking fit and feeling great. Whether we are trying to lose weight, just eat right, or build muscle, the smartest thing to do is create a healthy eating plan.

Primary goal: To lose weight or to build muscle

In order to lose weight we must consume fewer calories per day than our maintenance level amount. Doing so creates a caloric deficit which forces our body to start burning our stored body fat for energy. The most often recommended caloric deficit is about 20% below maintenance level.

For example, Muriel's estimated calorie maintenance level was 2107 calories per day, at the time we started. Her weight was 96 kg, 1.58 height, she was not all that active. 20% of 2107 is 421. We subtracted that 421 from 2107 and got 1686. Muriel needed to eat 1686 calories per day to lose fat. And so she did, approximately.

In order to build muscle, besides activating them with strength training, we must consume more calories per day than maintenance level. Doing so creates a caloric surplus, and this provides the body with the calories it needs to actually create new muscle tissue. A caloric surplus, combined with strength exercise, is a muscle-building requirement. The ideal caloric surplus for most men is about 250 calories above maintenance level, and around half that for women.

For example, Matt started our health process with an estimated calorie maintenance level of ~2400 calories per day. His weight was 94, 1.82 and he was definitely not very active. Had his goal been to build muscles tissue at an ideal rate he would have needed to add 250 to 2400 and eat about 2650 calories per day.

Oliver, the former hypotonic kid who is now a 15 year-old young man just set a new goal in the Gymind process, that is, to build his muscles. He is currently very thin, weighing 61 kg on 1.75. He plays tennis twice a week, occasionally shoots hoops with friends, and trains with me at the studio: weight lifting, cycling training, step aerobics, etc. For him, it is important to eat his 2310 kcal. per day.

Weigh yourself once a week first thing in the morning before you eat or drink, making sure your weight is moving in the right direction at the optimal rate. If your goal is losing weight, you should end up losing between 0.2-0.8 grams per week, closer to 1 kilo if you have a lot of fat to lose, closer to 0.2 grams if you only have a little fat to lose, or somewhere in the middle if you have an average amount to lose. If your goal is to build muscle, you should end up gaining about 0.2 grams per week (or about 1 kilo per month). If you are consistently gaining weight faster than that, reduce your calorie intake by about 250 calories. If you are gaining weight slower than that or not at all, then increase your calorie intake by about 250 calories.

The most common recommendation for the daily protein intake of healthy adults who are weight training regularly is between 0.8 - 1.5 grams of protein per one kilogram of body weight. An even 1 gram of protein per kilo is probably the most common recommendation of all. Protein is the key nutrient for building muscle. Men, especially in their 20s, should nevertheless take in at least 30 percent of their total calories from high-quality protein sources like lean meats, fish, dairy, poultry, eggs or egg whites, milk, protein supplements, nuts, and beans (Treyzon, 2008). To speed recovery from power workouts, drink a shake made with at least 20 grams of whey protein powder, 1/3 cup milk, 1 cup cranberry juice, and 1 cup frozen mixed berries (which are inflammation fighters).

Fat should account for between 20-30% of your total calorie intake, with an even 25 % probably being most common. 1 gram of fat contains 9 calories.

For example, Muriel's ideal calorie intake started with 1686 calories per day. 25% of 1686 is 421. Dividing 421 by 9 shows that Muriel needs to eat about 46.8 grams of fat per day.

Fat will not make you fat (Zinczenko, 2010). In fact, not eating enough fat can make you fat. A 2008 study published in the New England Journal of medicine found that a diet high in healthy fats proves to be superior to a low-fat diet, both in terms of weight loss and overall health benefits. (Eckel, 2008). Saturated and trans fat have given fat a bad reputation, but the truth is that the unsaturated fats found in foods like nuts, seeds, salmon, and olive oil are key components of a healthy diet.

Basically, figure out how many calories your protein and fat intake will account for, and then subtract them from your ideal total calorie intake. The majority of your carb intake should come from foods like fruits and vegetables, rice, sweet potatoes, white potatoes, and various beans and whole wheat or whole grain products.

The low carb craze of the early 2000s had people terrified of breaking bread, but eating the right kinds of breads and other grains can actually help you lose weight. An American Journal of Clinical Nutrition study found that people who obtained most of their grain servings from whole grains had less belly fat than those who skipped the whole grains (Katcher, 2008). The reason: The fiber found in whole grain foods helps slow digestion, keeping you fuller longer. You should still avoid refined grains like "enriched" flour, but a moderate amount of whole grain bread can be a great addition to a balanced diet (Zinczenko, 2013).

Muriel's nutrition plan, step by step

We know now that at the time she began the Gymind process, Muriel weighed 96 kg. and needed a calorie deficit in order to reach her goal, i.e., to eat 1686 calories per day. We trained together (and still do) twice a week, so we predicted a higher maintenance level and a weight-loss at a good pace.

We also know that she needs to eat about 46.8 grams of fat per day, or 421 kcal. from fat.

We decided to go with an even 0.8 grams of protein per kilo of body weight. Since she weighs 96 kg., that means she needed to eat about 76.8 grams of protein per day. Since 1 gram of protein contains 4 calories, that means her protein intake will account for 307.2 calories each day.

At this point, Muriel has 307.2 calories worth of protein and 421 calories worth of fat, which means a total of 728.2 of her daily calorie intake is accounted for. Since she should be eating 1686 calories per day she has 957.8 calories that are not yet accounted for.

Those 957.8 calories will come from carbs. Since 1 gram of carbs contains 4 calories, Muriel needed to eat about 239.5 grams of carbs per day.

Muriel needed:

1686 kcal per day

46.8 grams of fat per day

76.8 grams of protein per day

239.5 grams of carbs per day

7:00: 150 kcal, 4 grams of fat, 6 grams of protein, 21 grams of carbs: 1 glass of chocolate milk.

10:30: 360 kcal, 15.3+ 0.9+0.3 grams of fat, 1.7+5.7+1.8 grams of protein, 5+29.4+9 grams of carbs: 2 slices of whole wheat bread with half an avocado and red pepper.

12:30: 500 kcal, 1.1+4.5+ 0.2 grams of fat, 4.8+43.5+3.6 grams of protein, 49.7+0+ 7.3 grams of carbs: Brown rice, chicken breast 150 grams, peas, or humus.

15:00: 200 kcal: 0+1.6 grams of fat, 0+ 3.9 grams of protein, 19.3+ 30 grams of carbs: Popsicle and a cup of whole wheat bagels.

17:00: 150 kcal: 0.2+0.5grams of fat ,0.1+ 1grams of protein, 9.9+

21.5 grams of carbs: An apple and a banana.

19:30: 400 kcal, 12.1+14+2.5 grams of fat, 14.3+0+ 5.2 grams of protein, 1.2+0+0.7 grams of carbs: 2 scrambled eggs, a salad with a tbsp. of olive oil, 2 tbsp. of cottage cheese.

According to this example of Muriel's nutrition plan:

Total of 1760 kcal

Total of grams 57.2 of fat

Total of 91.6 grams of protein

Total of 203 grams of carbs

That's how we ensured that Muriel ate the right number of calories each day along with an optimal amount of protein, fat, and carbs that ideally come mostly from high quality sources.

Muriel's clever attitude

Snacking throughout the day is actually one of the best ways to avoid an expanding waistline. In a recent study conducted in Alabama, researchers discovered that people who snacked four or more times a day took in fewer calories and had lower BMIs than those who did not snack at all. (Wroten, 2012). Consistent snacking helps maintain blood sugar level, curbs cravings, and prevents the body from storing excess fat. The most effective snacks are high in protein and low in sugar. Two great options are nuts and low-fat dairy products. (Zinczenko, 2013).

Once we constructed Muriel's nutrition plan, we just had to make it as suitable and as comfortable as possible, in order to help Muriel embrace this healthy life-style for good.

Muriel LOVES to eat; she enjoys good foods and appreciates them. A great meal with friends at least once a week is a must. In line with that, when some foods are not all that tasty for her, she should not eat them. Muriel has a sweet tooth; she could take a chocolate bar that was not very fresh but eat it anyway "just 'cause it's there" as she said. No more.

Muriel is a manager at a gas station which also sells food. She is surrounded by temptations and endless fattening opportunities that got her into this weight problem in the first place. Night snacks were welcomed for Muriel who occasionally finishes work late at night.

Had we decided to completely change Muriel's life-style, her health process probably wouldn't last that long and she would have soon gone back to being heavy and inactive.

Muriel occasionally contacted me from work, asking about calories in the spirit of "Should I?"; "Is this ok to munch now?"; "Does this product contain less than 100 calories?"

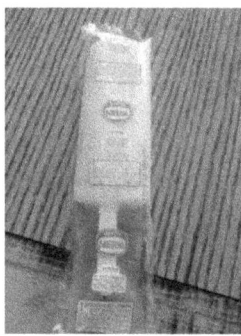

Muriel sends me a picture and "gets permission" to enjoy a 67-calorie Popsicle.

So we integrated her healthy nutrition plan with a calorie deficit and got ourselves one happy 22 year-old girl who, 5 years later, still enjoys her nice figure and her health.

Muriel's interaction with "Plateau"

Muriel began to lose weight at a very impressive rate. This is a segment of her progress chart:

Day	Kg	Loss
Aug 31st 2008	88.7 1.62	R arm 39 cm Belly 101 R thigh 69
Sep 6th 2008	85.5	3.2☺ ☺
Sep 13th 2008	84.3	1.2 ☺ ☺
Sep 20th 2008	84.4	R 34.5 Belly 101
Sep 30th 2008	82.3	R. thigh 62 :
October 4th 2008	81.8	Belly 95
October 18th 2008	79.4	
November 2nd 2008	77.5	☺☺☺new t shirt size M
November 16th 2008	74.5	L 31 Thigh 59 Belly 89
December 9th	71.7	R30 Thigh 59 Belly 90

When we hit 71 kilograms, Muriel's weight was "stuck" on that number. We changed the math equation for calorie deficit, we created changes in physical activity, but nothing helped, and Muriel stayed at that weight for over 6 months (!) until the weight began to "move" again and in the right direction.

Studies show that resistance to further weight loss, what called a 'plateau', is a significant phenomenon in obese men subjected to a weight-reducing program (Tremblay, 2009). These plateaus occur because it's a biological inevitability when we continue to constantly restrict calories. The less we eat, the more our metabolism starts to slow down. It's a survival mechanism: the body thinks that food is becoming scarce, so in an effort to survive, it starts to use energy more efficiently. As a result, our fat loss requires an even further caloric restriction. So we eat even less, prompting our body to slow its metabolism down even more, again repeating the cycle. The Alpert theoretical paper (2005) suggests that there is a physiological limit to how fast we can burn or lose fat. If we try to force the body with huge deficits, then beyond a certain point the composition of the weight loss would shift to more lean body mass and less fat. This study supports the idea that the overweight and obese can safely use a larger deficit and lose more fat while the already lean who want to get leaner need to lose fat more slowly or they risk muscle loss.

Weight loss until the point of resistance to further weight loss may be detrimental for some psychobiological variables including depression when prescribing a weight reduction program for obese individuals. (Chaput, 2007). However, Muriel stayed positive. In an interview she gave the Israeli "Menta Health Magazine" back in September of 2012, she was quoted as saying: "I never set a definite target for myself, such as losing weight for a certain event at a certain time. I chose to address the whole process as a way of life. So when I hit plateaus during the Gymind process, it was ok, it was part of the deal".

For Muriel, psychologically speaking, the weight is not the goal. Going on the right path to health certainly is.

Muriel embraced the thought that this is her new life-style, that this is the right path for her, and she enjoys her life as it is. Muriel learned the lesson of patience. Losing weight should be a process, a long one, a way of life. Muriel was "forced" to accept that this is her new way now, for life. Then, when her body finally reached its ideal weight, Muriel could enjoy this weight for a long time, also enjoying her healthy-convenient life-style.

In Hebrew the word "wait" can also be interpreted as "the gift". In English the present time is also a "present". Muriel was obliged to accept the present for the way it is, a real present.

Successful Strategies for Long-Term Weight Loss Success

Successful weight loss maintenance has been defined as intentional weight loss of at least 10% of body weight, which is kept off for at least one year. This criterion has been established because weight loss of 10% of initial weight in overweight and obese persons is associated with meaningful reductions in the risk for heart disease and diabetes. (Wing and Phelan, 2005). Initial research on registry members by Klem and colleagues in 1997 uncovered three common strategies for successful weight loss maintenance that remained consistent in the 2005 findings:

Doing high levels of physical activity

Consuming a low-calorie, low-fat diet

Weighing oneself frequently

The 2005 study identified a fourth common strategy: most (78%) members reported eating breakfast (typically cereal and fruit) every day. This study also found that members ate 2.5 meals per week at a restaurant and 0.74 meals per week in fast-food establishments. A common trait that has been observed in successful weight losers is their vigilance regarding weight loss maintenance. Wing and Phelan (2005) noted that more than 44% of registry members weighed themselves daily, while 31% weighed themselves at least once per week. Further investigation revealed that "successful weight loss maintainers continue to act like recently successful weight losers for many years after their weight loss".
Engaging in high levels of physical activity each week is also common among those who maintain long-term weight loss. In the 2005 study, men reported an average physical activity expenditure of 3,293 kcal per week and women an average of 2,545 kcal per week. This level of physical activity is equivalent to about one hour per day of moderate-intensity activity. Previous research showed that as registry members decreased their physical activity by more than 800 kcal per week, there was a tendency to regain some weight (McGuire, 1999).

Why do some people remain slimmer than others? The answer may be in the amount of time lean individuals spend fidgeting, standing, and walking around compared with sitting still (Ravussin, 2005). Animal and human studies suggest that individual levels of spontaneous physical activity are inherent and biologically regulated, and high levels may protect against obesity and gaining back weight (Kotz, 2008).

Some thoughts about "Menu fit all"

My continuing work for so many years with wonderful individuals who are taking care of themselves throughout their search for health yields some thoughts about the right nutrition for all mankind. Just like the axiomatic information about how walking is good for your health, how strength training in important for your muscles, and how much stretching is a must for your joints and your soul, there is some solid evidence as far as "eating smart" is concerned adequate for healthy people who wish to optimize their body potential now and for a long time. Or as Agin, (2008), in his "light" yet scholarly approach puts it: Your body needs continuous respect and appreciation and if treated well can provide a wonderful healthy life.

Listen to your needs:

Oprah (2004, the Oprah magazine) talks about the belief she has about eating well: "I know for sure that a meal that brings you real pleasure will do you more good in the long and short term than a lot of "filler" food that leaves you standing in your kitchen, roaming from cabinet to fridge. I call it that grazing feeling: You want something but can't figure out what it is. All the carrots, celery, and skinless chicken in the world can't give you the satisfaction of one good piece of chocolate if that's what you really crave".

Breakfast is important:

Even if we don't have time to sit down and enjoy a peaceful breakfast in the morning, this is still the most important meal of the day. There are plenty of grab-and-go ways to start your day. A low-fat yogurt is a great choice, but don't forget to pair it with a handful of unsalted nuts for extra protein and a dose of "good" fat. Take a banana or other easy-to-grab fruit and add an energy bar that has no more than 100 calories.

Plan, get fully equipped for the day:

The best way to eat smart throughout the day is to plan. Even if you're not a super-organized person, just taking 10 minutes to make a weekly shopping list full of healthy foods is guaranteed to keep you on the healthy eating track. Keep a box of instant oatmeal at work. (All you need is a microwave and you're all set for an energized morning), some apples and dates in your bag. Come what may – a meeting, a long day with a restaurant out of sight - you will always have a nutritious snack to eat every 2 hours. It will keep you focused and energetic.

At dinner time:

It's so easy to order pizza or Chinese takeout, but try to keep it to a minimum. If you haven't gotten in your five to nine servings of fruits and vegetables for the day, make an extra effort to include them now.

Choose them right:

Over the years we have collected a grocery list of the most important ingredients we should all consume daily. To satisfy hunger, to get the entire nutrients our body needs: An apple a day, a handful of nuts, an egg, 40 grams of dark chocolate (40% cacao), 10-14 cups of water.

Awareness, Responsibility and changing the "Automaton"

One of the most unwise dieting tricks ever is the idea of distracting yourself to keep from eating: "think about other things, anything that will get your mind off of food. According to Dutch research, thinking about snacks and meals can actually help you stay lean. The study found that when asked questions like "what will you do if you get hungry 2 hours before your next meal?", thinner participants were better able to give healthy responses, like "eat a handful of nuts". (Glanz, 1997). Taking a proactive approach to your diet by thinking ahead will help you stay thin (Zinczenko, 2013).

Belle stepped on the scale and did not like what she saw: "74.5? How is it possible?" She complained. "I did everything right this week only to see I gained 200 grams?" Belle was not expecting her period, (which may make her feel somewhat bloated), and she was more active this week. "Tell me what you ate today, yesterday, and the day before" I said. "Something must have been different". After long contemplation Belle suddenly remembered: "Saturday night, at home, without even noticing, automatically I would say, Leroy and I ate salty roasted nuts, half a kilo. WOW. That's amazing. I don't think I was even aware of that".

That automatic behavior represents the fact the "someone else is riding the bus" as Bandler (1974) stated; the subconscious mind is in action, overshadowing the conscious "lucid judgment". We act upon something without thinking, without giving it much notice. And we pay a price.

"I now understand this whole thing about the automatic behavior," Simone[4] called me one day, enthusiastic. "I was just at Safeway, doing my grocery shopping as usual, when I realized I was eating a bag of chips I just took from the shelf. I stopped immediately but it was definitely an automatic behavior of mine".

Belle and Simone's stories are representative of most of our everyday "behaviors". In the previous chapter we called it "a habit", dealing with the question of how to change a bad habit. The continued growth of the obesity epidemic at a time when obesity is highly

4 Simone, 22, went through the Gymind Process in California. Simone's goal was to lose the weight in order to wear the perfect wedding dress. From size 14 she became a size 8.

stigmatized should make us question the assumption that, given the right information and motivation, people can successfully reduce their food intake over the long term. It does not seem to be that simple. Automatic behaviors are those that occur without awareness, are initiated without intention, tend to continue without control, and operate efficiently or with little effort. The concept that eating is an automatic behavior is supported by studies that demonstrate the impact of the environmental context and food presentation on eating (Cohen, 2008). The amount of food eaten is strongly influenced by factors such as portion size, food visibility, and the ease of obtaining food. Moreover, people are often unaware of the amount of food they have eaten or of the environmental influences on their eating. A revised view of eating as an automatic behavior, as opposed to one that humans can self-regulate, has profound implications for our response to the obesity epidemic, suggesting that the focus should be less on nutrition education and more on shaping the food environment.

I often tell my clients about the "inner elevator" we possess inside our body and how moving the elevator up toward our head or down into our guts can create a behavior. When the voice of reason calms down a certain emotion or takes charge over a profound deep habit, then our elevator moves DOWN to convey a message and makes us act upon it. It moves UP when a certain habit or an Automat takes control. The more we are aware of that dialogue between UP and DOWN, the more we listen to our body, the more we are at ease with ourselves: less "taken by surprise" and more in control. Researchers show how cognitive change contributes to symptom change (Teachmen, 2008).

"3 minutes", I said once at a seminar held in Tel-Aviv. "That's the difference between a fat person and a thin person". How come? In 3 minutes we can automatically eat thousands of calories, (a doughnut, 500 kcal, a slice of pizza, 450 kcal, a chocolate bar, 500 kcal), no more than 3 minutes, that's how long it takes. But if we stop for a second and convert those 3 minutes with 3 seconds of an inner dialogue: Am I hungry? What do I really need to eat now? that makes all the difference. We would probably not continue to eatithose thousands of calories.

Read nutrition labels for better health

The Nutrition Labeling and Education Act of 1990 mandated that standardized nutrition information appear on almost all packaged foods manufactured after May 1994. Reading and understanding nutrition labels on foods may be an important precursor to dietary change (Kreuter, 1997). The relationship between label use and diet is clear now: the Cancer Prevention Research Program in Seattle found that people successfully limited their fat intake by making use of nutrition labels (Neuhouser, 1999). The Division of Epidemiology and Community Health at the University of Minnesota states that individuals who frequently read nutrition labels tend to both value healthy eating and to engage in healthy dietary practices more than individuals who read labels infrequently. However, the relationship between label use, attitude toward healthy eating, and dietary quality remains unclear, particularly among young adults, about whom little is known with regard to nutrition label use. In fact, a study found that nutrition label reading does not translate into a healthier diet in adolescents (Huang, 2004).

The Minnesota study investigated whether nutrition label use mediates the relationship between eating-related attitudes and dietary behaviors among young adult college students. Students who reported frequently reading nutrition labels were more likely to have healthier dietary intakes (less fast food and added sugar; more fiber, fruits, and vegetables) compared to those who read labels sometimes or rarely. Further, frequent nutrition label use was a significant partial mediator of the relationship between eating-related attitudes (feeling that it is important to prepare healthy meals) and dietary quality, indicating that label use may be one means by which individuals who value healthy eating translate their attitude into healthy eating behaviors. Even among those who did not believe it was important to prepare healthy meals, frequent nutrition label use was significantly associated with healthier dietary intake, suggesting that label use may operate independently of nutrition-related attitude in contributing to a healthful diet (Graham, 2012).

Washington State University economist Bidisha Mandal found that middle-aged Americans who want to lose weight and who take up the label-reading habit are more likely to lose weight than those who don't. In some cases, label reading is even more effective than exercise. "People who are trying to lose weight want to know what they're buying and preparing, and many do better if they use labels to find what they need to know," she says. Writing in the latest Journal of Consumer Affairs, Mandal analyzes the responses of more than 3,700 people who regularly took a national survey asking about their label-reading habits while attempting to lose or control their weight. Among her findings:

If you want to lose weight, you have a better chance of success if you read a food label when you first buy a product.

People are more successful at losing weight when they add label reading to their exercise program.

Label readers who do not exercise have a slightly greater chance of losing weight than those who exercise but do not read labels.

Women are more likely to read food labels when they buy a product for the first time, possibly because they are responsible for buying food and cooking. They are also more successful than men in losing weight.

Become a "critic consumer," I told Tom, the 12-year-old girl. When you're shopping with your mom, try to read food labels, to compare brands. Turn the product upside down and look at the list of ingredients. It gives you a lot of information and information means power, being in control, being in charge. Check the Nutrition Facts tables to compare serving sizes, nutrient amounts and % DV. Choose foods that have more vitamins, minerals, and fiber, and less fat, sodium, and sugar.

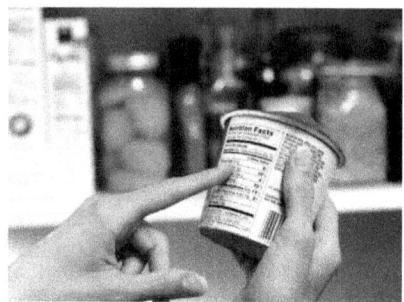

Reading food labels (in http://wellbeingmagazine.co.uk/)

Take a picture, take charge, and take care

One of the Gymind methods to help take charge over the inner elevator is to take a picture of your dish. Clients send me a picture and receive a "calorie pricing" that enables them to continue planning the rest of their day, calorie-wise. But more so, it forces them to stop for "3 seconds", to take charge, and avoid those "fattening 3 minutes" they need to stay away from.

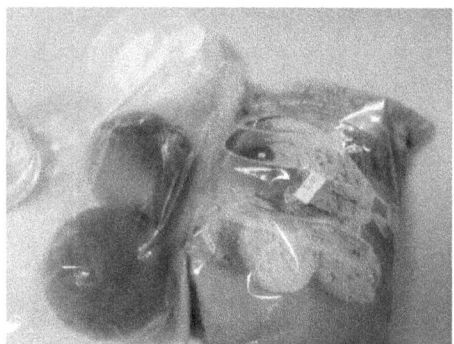

Tami's Lunch box for school: Honey rice crispers, two peaches, 2 tbsp. of cottage cheese: 380 kcal.

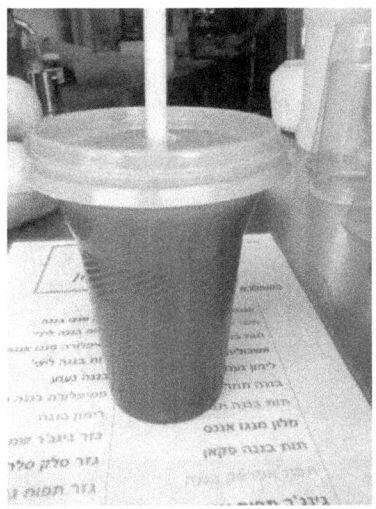

Irene's healthy morning drink: Beet, carrot, apple, and celery: 100 kcal.

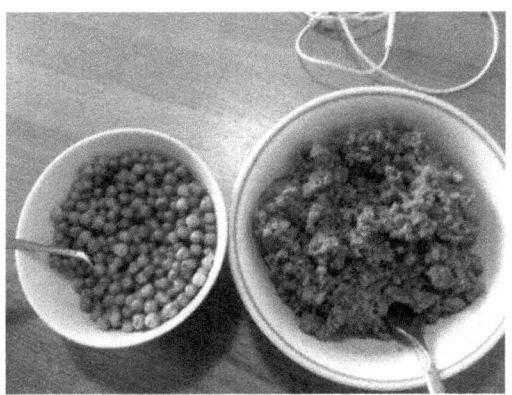

A bowl of peas and a bowl of ground beef for lunch: ~ 450 kcal.

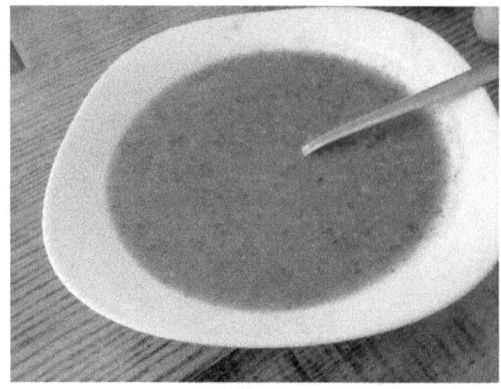

A bowl of lentil soup: 150 kcal.

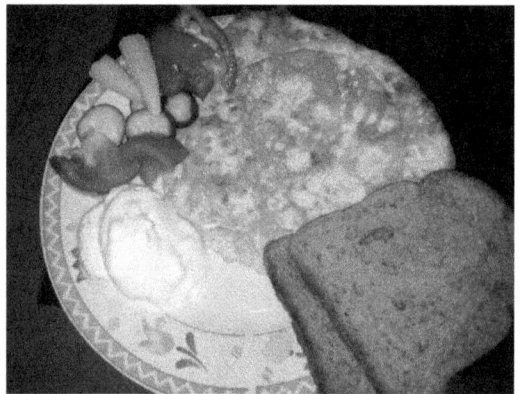

A nutritious breakfast of approximately 250 kcal.

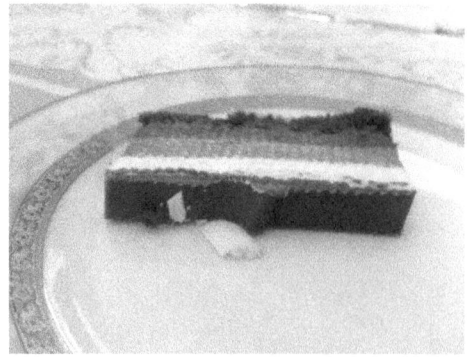

Aida's idea of a "happy dish" once a week: 350 kcal.

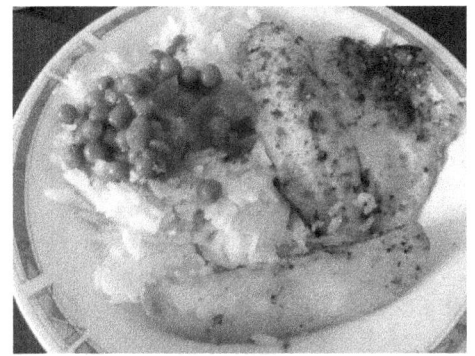

Rice, peas, potato, and chicken: 350 kcal.

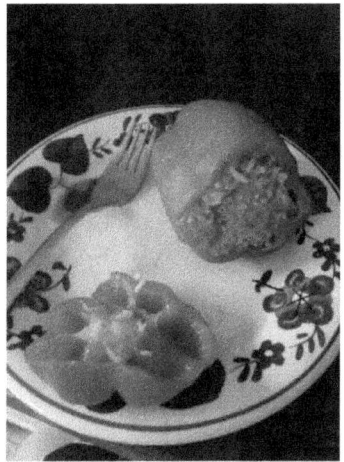

Stuffed red pepper, with meat and rice: 200 kcal.

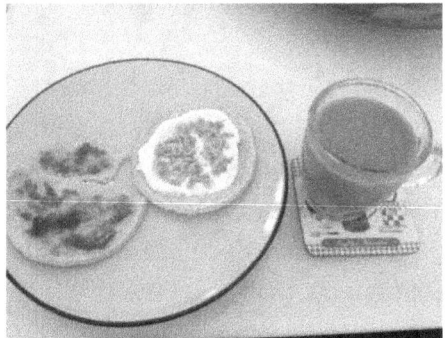

Irene's breakfast: Wheat crispers with tuna and cheese, one with jam, coffee: 150 kcal.

Can we change the automaton?

We would start with a straight answer: Oh yes, we can. We can change the inner compass we have had since childhood that we might have forgotten all about.

Just like with breathing: Look at a baby's breath. His stomach goes up and down. His pulse is higher than that of a grown up yet he manages to breathe deep into his belly. As years go by, our breath gets more flat: Into the lungs, then through our nose and then we sometimes "forget to breathe". A constant reminder and proper practice would help us go back to our roots as "deep breathers". This baby who takes an "automatic deep breath" asks for food only when he feels the need to eat. And when he's done, he does not eat more than he should. Somewhere along the way, distracted by so many elements, his mom is trying to feed him "because there are hungry children in Somalia"; portion sizes that are big enough; food visibility that invites you to "eat me"; ease of obtaining affordable foods; social eating; emotional eating. It's that comforting large piece of chocolate cake that automatically and subconsciously brings you back to your birthday parties from your childhood and eases the pain. Can we change that? Can we go back to our natural, pure needs as babies?

Several ways were found to be mostly effective, and they have everything to do with dialoging with the subconscious. Recent studies found that Cognitive Behavioral Therapy (CBT) is an effective treatment for emotional disorders such as anxiety or depression. Cognitive behavioral therapy rapidly affects automatic processing, and these early effects are predictive of later therapeutic change. Such results suggest very fast action on automatic processes mediating threat sensitivity, providing an early marker of treatment response. Furthermore, these findings challenge the notion that psychological treatments work directly on conscious thought processes before automatic information processing and imply a greater similarity between early effects of pharmacological and psychological treatments for anxiety than previously though. (Reinecke, 2013). It's also training in the Neuro-Linguistic Programming techniques, (NLP), of shifting perceptual position, visual-kinesthetic dissociation, timelines, and change-history, all based on experiential cognitive processing of remembered events that leads to an increased awareness of behavioral contingencies and a more sensitive recognition of environmental cues which could serve to lower anxiety and increase the sense of internal control (Kunefal, 1992). We will discuss all that in chapter 3 when dealing with the MIND and SPIRIT. For now, some powerful and specific "fit all" techniques to help create a change of the automaton.

Like to dislike; the NLP technique

Can you think of something that you like but wish you did not? Good, what is it? As you think about it, do you have a picture? (Elicit Submodalities: Visual, Auditory, Kinesthetic. For example: How does it look? Where is it located? How do you feel about it?). Let's say you wish you did not like ice cream. □

Can you think of something which is similar, but which you absolutely dislike? For example, yoghurt. (Elicit the SubModalities. The location of both pictures should be different).

Change the SubModalities of #1 into the SubModalities of #2.

Lock it in place. "You know the sound that Tupperware makes when it seals. Just like that, lock it right there".

Now, what about that thing you used to like?
How is it different now?

Future Pace: "Imagine a time in the future when you might be tempted to eat ice-cream. What happens now?"

Beware of "non-ecological" shifts

We encounter this phenomenon mostly with kids who won't try to eat vegetables; kids who "decide" this one day, or since always have been reluctant to try vegetables, fruits or certain foods other than pizza, pasta, mac & cheese or burgers. Despite considerable epidemiological evidence of the health benefits of a diet high in fruit and vegetables, consumption by pre-school children remains well below recommended levels. Children's consumption of fruit and vegetables are related to different psychosocial and environmental factors. Promotion of this behavior may require attention to nutritional education and child-feeding strategies of parents. (Gibson, 1998). A cancer research from London evaluated the effectiveness of an exposure-based intervention, carried out by parents in the home, for increasing children's liking for a previously disliked vegetable. It concluded (Wardle, 2003) that a parent-led, exposure-based intervention involving daily tasting of a vegetable holds promise for improving children's acceptance of vegetables. Apparently a "Dislike to Like" technique should change that "automaton" rejection for the better, easily enabling children to eat or better yet, even "like" vegetables. However, this shift must be ecological. That is, if a child refuses to eat a certain legume it might be because he is allergic to it and does not know it. His subconscious mind may know the reason for that refusal and "protects" the body from eating a certain nutrient, no matter how "healthy for you" it is considered to be "by others". Bottom line, we can change the automaton, but we should first listen to our inner compass as to whether it's the right thing for us to do.

This "automatic eating" is related to studies on "intuitive eating", which is eating based on feelings of hunger and fullness rather than on emotions or situations. The focus on intuitive eating is an attempt to find out what constitutes healthy eating, rather than the more prevalent focus in psychology on eating disorders. Many people can't believe people should be able to eat when they want and whatever foods they want. There's a belief that if you give people unconditional permission to eat, they are going to binge and add a lot of kilograms. But that's not necessarily the case. A study of 199 college women, published in April 2007 in the Journal of Counseling Psychology, found that those who followed intuitive eating principles actually had a slightly lower body mass index (BMI) than women who did not. If you listen to your body signals in determining what, when, and how much to eat, you are not going to binge, and you're going to eat an appropriate amount of nutrient-dense foods (Tylka, 2007).

Children's Nutrition, at home and at school: Regulations and recommendations

Obesity among children affects their physical development, body image, and self-confidence and may break their spirit. However, the statistics from all over the world do not paint a bright picture. The 1992 Bogalusa Heart Study[5] confirmed the existence of fatty plaques and streaks, (the beginning of atherosclerosis), in most children and teenagers. (Berenson, 2001). Public health efforts to improve the obesity-related behaviors of US adolescents may be having some success (Ronald, 2012), but children all over the world are heavier than in the past (Hatav, 1998). Eating should be enjoyable, but it should also serve to keep kids and students looking fit and feeling great. So, change for the better begins at home and at school. By learning about the importance of the various macronutrient groups, (carbohydrates, proteins, and fats), and the value of information in nutrition labels, children are better educated to make informed choices about eating, so fad diets begin to lose their appeal as long-term options. (May, 2012) Children, according to Dr. Oz, should "give parents a hard time" so they all live better. Because most children do not normally think about health issues, adults have to communicate either directly or indirectly through the behaviors they enact. Parents will not let children sit around the table smoking cigarettes and drinking whiskey, because it is not socially acceptable, but is it fine to let them consume cola, fries cooked in trans-fat, and a cheeseburger regularly? Many children consume doughnuts, cookies,

---

5 The Bogalusa Heart Study began in 1972 as an epidemiology study of cardiovascular risk factors in children and adolescents; it eventually evolved into observations of young adults (Berenson, 2001).

cupcakes, and candy on a daily basis (Fuhrman, 2003).

A study published in the Health Education Research states that a positive parental role model may be a better method for improving a child's diet than attempts at dietary control. (Brown, 2004). Another British study found that family mealtime is related to dietary quality and intake (Sweetman, 2011). Parents can set standards for the kinds of foods their children are eating and help them develop healthy eating behaviors (Salvy, 2012). There is some evidence that family-based behavior modification programs, where parents take primary responsibility and act as "agents of change", may help children to lose weight (Wilson, 2003).

Provide healthier food at home.

Remove the bad foods from the house and "don't invite any enemies" to come in.

Expose kids to a variety of healthier food options.

Studies support the idea that a breakfast with a lower sugar load may improve short-term memory and attention span at school (Benton, 2007). Giving your child a breakfast which contains fiber, (oatmeal, shredded wheat, berries, bananas, whole-grain pancakes, etc.), instead of loads of refined sugar should keep adrenaline levels more constant and make the school day a more pleasant and productive experience.

Work with the parents of your child's friends to create better eating habits for your child and his friends. When the eating habit change occurs in one of the friends or in both of the friends, it's more likely to be maintained because the kids reinforce each other in those healthy behaviors.

Get your child involved with other friends. Kids are more physically active when they are with other kids. They don't run on treadmills; they play with their friends. That's how they get their physical activities.

Researchers at the University of Buffalo in New York observed 23 overweight and 42 "non-overweight" children who were given the opportunity to play and eat with a friend or with a peer they didn't know. The results of the study showed that the overweight children who ate with their overweight friends consumed more food than when they were with thinner children or children who weren't their friends. The overweight children ate more because their friends influenced them to increase their food intake (Temple, 2008). This study's results reflect a child's need to feel accepted by other children. Although family has a huge impact on food and making foods available, kids are spending a lot of time with their friends, peers at school, and on sports teams. As they get older, the more influence their friends and peers have. The research also highlights the benefits of friendship. Friends can also help each other become healthier. It's not about forbidding kids to eat with overweight kids, but it is about changing the friends' habits so they're actually reinforcing each other's habits.

A Dutch study, (Tak, 2010), provides some evidence that the Schoolgruiten intervention effect on fruit and vegetable intake also reduced unhealthy snacking during school breaks. The goal of another Dutch study was to investigate the relative importance of personal and social environmental predictors of the consumption of fruit, high-fat snacks, and breakfast (Martens 2005). The results indicate that adolescents' attitudes are the most important determinants of different health-related eating behaviors and intentions to change. Interventions promoting a healthy diet for adolescents should include creative strategies to achieve positive associations with healthy dietary changes. The Child and Adolescent Trial for Cardiovascular Health tested the effectiveness of a multilevel intervention aimed at promoting a healthful school environment and positive eating and physical activity behaviors in children. They targeted the school food service staff and aimed to lower the total fat, saturated fat, and sodium content of school meals (Osganian, 1996).

Adolescence is a time when boys and girls can gain or lose significant amounts of weight, both of which can have harmful effects on health. It's a difficult time for this age group because they have more flexibility in food choices and may be drawn towards fast food, containing lots of saturated fat which can lead to obesity. Faddy diets are often shared among pupils at school, putting teenagers at risk of deficiencies in micro-nutrients such as calcium, B vitamins, and iron. It can also lead to eating disorders which increase the risk of osteoporosis in later life. According to the National Diet and Nutrition Survey (2009), approximately 40 percent of teenagers have low iron stores which can result in a lack of energy and absence of menstrual periods in girls.

A study from the Hebrew University in Jerusalem concluded that over the long term, treatment of childhood obesity with the parents as the exclusive agents of change was superior to the conventional approach (Golan, 2004).

Liana's nutrition plan, supported by her family

We remember Liana, the 4-year-old girl, so sweet yet so heavy, who was obliged to engage in physical activity in order to lose weight. Now at the age of 6 Liana is much stronger. She recently confided to me that "exercise is fun" (that was a huge WOW moment), yet that same exciting notion was followed by a genuine request for some juice and snacks. Other clients who visit the studio at the following hour are almost always amazed to see a sweet girl holding a bag of potato chips or a chocolate bar that Liana has brought to our session. "Something is wrong with that picture," they say with a kind smile. Liana is "attached" to that bag of chips or that chocolate bar, does not necessarily eat them, yet receives some comfort and maybe also achieve a sense of control just by holding them.

Her parents are very much involved. They have fully understood by now that changes must be done at home and that grocery shopping will not be the same. What has changed?

Indeed, they still buy potato chips and chocolate bars, but less than before. Some snacks do not enter the house: Cookies, certain salty snacks, for example, are out of the equation. Pop-corn, Bamba, (an Israeli peanut snack), and small, plain 67 calorie chocolate bars are ok to consume. That's it.

Portions became much smaller. Liana's mom sets out meals on smaller plates to make the portion on the plate look bigger. Liana can't give up hot-dogs, so instead of eating 4 of them as usual her mom takes two hot-dogs and slices the hot-dog lenghthwise, placing 4 halves on the plate which look like 4 whole hot-dogs. Half the calories, half the sodium.

Disposable cups usually made for soft drinks serve as a holder for snacks and cornflakes. For example: For an afternoon snack, Liana would take a disposable cup and fill it with 30 grams of cheerios.

Limitations and new rules: Two chocolate bars and one disposable cup for snacks, (popcorn or potato chips) a day. No French fries at restaurants and no saturated foods whatsoever. The key word at home is "health", for everybody.

Eating slowly: This may be one of the most important things Liana has engaged herself to since embracing the Gymind process. Eating slowly. Chewing food properly. Enjoying every bite in the mouth and helping digestion take its course from the beginning point making a perfect use of saliva enzymes. We used as a method the Erikson personifications and Metaphor, (Rosen 1991), as a path to Liana's subconscious mind: "The food in your mouth is your best friend playing with you, wishing to stay with you for as much as he could, tickling you, holding you. Let him be there for as long as it needs to". Liana's chewing and swallowing behavior has changed dramatically.

At some point throughout the process, maybe the break-through moment, was when Liana's 2 bothers joined the Gymind process. Matt and Dan, (15, 11), who both had been gaining 10 extra kilograms and needed to lose weight, play a significant role in Liana's life as two older brothers to admire and worship. Liana spends long hours in the afternoon with Matt and Dan who had been having some difficulties in saying "no" to chocolate, candies, and unhealthy drinks when Liana asks for them, before engaging to the Gymind process. Now, once they fully understand the importance of eating smart and exercising, they feel stronger about setting limits and directing Liana to make the right choices.

Nutrition plan for kids who don't eat vegetables

Liana is a veggie hater. She will not eat broccoli, carrots, apples, nor even grapes. Although we know not to force her, nor to create an inner automatic change, we do want Liana to be exposed to vegetables. Her parents should offer her to try, and set a role model of a family who eats healthy nutrients. Even though Liana might resist vegetables now, maybe when she grows older her attitude might change.

In any case, concealing vegetables in food dishes, such as mashed carrots hidden in meat balls or shopped broccoli hidden in the Bolognese sauce, is a decent choice as long as you don't lie about it. A study published in the Journal of Nutrition Education and Behavior found that kids will happily eat baked goods that contain vegetables, even when they know there are veggies in the dough. Researchers served zucchini chocolate-chip bread, broccoli gingerbread spice cake, and chickpea chocolate-chip cookies to groups of schoolchildren. Kids liked the zucchini and broccoli treats, and only vetoed the chickpea cookies because they were unfamiliar with chickpeas (Pope, 2012).

Liana's mom received some new nutritious recipes that contain vegetables and other healthy nutrients, such as white rice mixed with hidden quinoa, humus beans in a shepherds' pie, and only tells Liana that those healthy ingredients are there somewhere.

Recommendations on the Assessment, Prevention, and Treatment of Childhood Obesity

In 2005 the American Medical Association published its Recommendations on the Assessment, Prevention, and Treatment of Childhood Obesity. The committee offered the following recommendations:

Assessment:

Annual measurement of weight, height, and body mass index (BMI).

Underweight: Below 5th percentile

Healthy Weight: 5th – 84th percentile

Overweight: 85th – 94th percentile

Obesity: 95th percentile or above

Child's medical history

Parental obesity

Family medical history

Other health problems related to obesity

Dietary, physical activity, and other behaviors

Prevention – Patient Level:

Limit	Encourage
Sugar-sweetened beverages TV/other screen time (no more than 2 hr/d) Eating out/restaurants Portion sizes Energy-dense (high calorie) foods	Fruits and vegetables: 9 servings/day Breakfast every day Family meals Physical activity (60 min/d of moderate to vigorous activity) Calcium Fiber Balanced fat, protein, carbohydrate intake for age Breastfeeding

Prevention – Practice and Community Level:

Increase physical activity at schools (grade 1 through college)

Preserve and enhance parks, walking, and bicycle paths

Encourage physicians and health professionals to support parents:

Authoritative (not restrictive) parenting style

As role models for healthy eating, physical activity, and reduced sedentary activities

Treatment:

Goal: improve long-term health through permanent healthy lifestyle habits

Stages

Prevention "Plus"
More frequent physician monitoring

Structured Weight Management
More specific goals and support to child

Comprehensive Multidisciplinary Intervention

Increased frequency of visits with more health providers

Tertiary Care Intervention
Medications, very low-calorie diets, and/or surgery for severely obese children

Oliver's Nutrition Plan

Oliver's eating habits have changed tremendously since he began the Gymind process. Indeed, he had always enjoyed healthy foods, thanks to his mother's awareness, but he still ate a lot, more than he needed, and he himself lacked the awareness and the responsibility for his body that a 12-year- old should feel. Luckily for him, Oliver drinks only water and he does not have a sweet tooth, so it was easy for him to give up sweets.

Oliver's daily nutrition plan:

Morning	A sandwich (two slices of bread, two tbsp. of white cheese or avocado or tahini sauce)
10:00	An apple or a banana or another nutritious sandwich
Lunch	A health portion of protein such as fish or chicken, a portion of nutritious carbs such as 6 tbsp. of brown rice or whole wheat pasta, vegetables
16:00	A cup of cottage cheese or a yogurt
Dinner	Vegetables, an egg, a piece of healthy pie.

(Brand-Miller, 2005)

Tami's Nutrition Plan

At the age of 12 and armed with a history of diets that did not yield much success with weight loss, Tami was very much aware of what she needed to eat and when. Smaller portions, healthier nutritious choices, less candies, less chocolate bars, and much more physical activity were all on the menu to boost up her metabolism. However, we did have to make some surprising adjustments along the way, since something seemed to be stuck. It was not the infamous plateau we had discussed earlier, since Tami never really lost a lot of weight and only then hit plateau. For months and months she grew stronger and felt better, without losing any fat. Indeed, the muscles she earned as a result of rope jumping, bicycle riding, and pedometer tracking contributed weight to her body, but still, we sensed that a fine-tuning of her nutrition was much needed.

We talked about how important whole grains were for her good health (Katcher, 2008), yet we decided to give up on them, especially wheat, (whole or white). Just as with celiac patients, we wanted to check to what extent Tami is in good terms with wheat products. The results were not long in coming, and during the weeks she did not consume gluten, Tami's weight moved in the right direction. A celiac blood test showed no sensitivity to gluten yet our small gluten-free trial showed that Tom's body is better off without it. Gluten sensitivity has been best recognized and understood in the context of two conditions, celiac disease and wheat allergy. However, according to a study from the Department of Gastroenterology in Oslo, some individuals complain of symptoms in response to ingestion of "gluten," without histologic or serologic evidence of celiac disease or wheat allergy. The term 'non-celiac gluten sensitivity' has been suggested for this condition, although a role for gluten proteins as the sole trigger of the associated symptoms remains to be established (Lundin, 2012). Future research is needed to generate more knowledge regarding non-celiac gluten sensitivity, a condition that has global acceptance but has only a few certainties and many unresolved issues. (Volta, 2013).

Tami eats whole wheat bread every now and then, but she mostly replaced pasta with rice, bread with rice crackers, and an energy bar made of granola with a chocolate bar or a popsicle.

Healthy body-Image and healthy eating

Body image is the picture that we have in our heads of what we look like (Varnado-Sullivan, 2004). Our physical health including our weight is by and large connected to the state of our emotions. Overweight and obesity are known to have a significant impact on psychological wellbeing developing a negative self-image, and experiencing low self-esteem. (Davison, 2001). Women who have a body image disturbance have a non-acceptance of their body size that often generalizes to their self-concept. (Stewart, 2004, 805). Women who accept their bodies the way they are seem to be more likely to follow principles of healthy eating (Tylk 2011), (Strauss 2000). When we feel good in our mind, this will translate to feeling good in our body, and vice versa. Success in every area of our life depends on how we see ourselves. When we truly believe in ourselves, we feel calmer, more centered, and more focused. Our metabolism starts working properly, our brain chemistry is balanced, and we don't need to reach for food to calm our emotions. In order to lose weight and keep it off, investing time in the pursuit of high self-esteem is in order. Reading. Studying. Meditating. Making a commitment to watch what we say to ourselves and about ourselves is so important. The words we use are so powerful (Austin, 1962), so we must refuse to engage in negative self-talk, and we should never give up on our body and mind.

Women's typical reason for changing their diet is dissatisfaction with their bodies. The message that women often hear is that some degree of body dissatisfaction is healthyn because it could help them strive to take care of their bodies. But it may be just the opposite. An appreciation of your body is needed to really adopt better eating habits (Tylk, 2011). A study from the Department of Psychology at Ohio State University found that women who reported they were intuitive eaters also reported higher levels of appreciation for their own body. They were more likely to agree with statements like "Despite its flaws, I accept my body for what it is". They were less likely to spend a lot of time thinking about how their body appears to others, and more time considering how their body feels and functions (Augustus-Horvath, 2011).

Meet Tamara and the needs of a lost 20-year-old

Tamara, 20, contacted me almost 10 years ago; disempowered, anxious and depressed. She was on a rollercoaster of self-punishment and failure. Tamara hated everything about herself (even though she was and still is one of the most beautiful girls I have encountered). She felt powerless and too weak to make changes in her body and soul. We had to treat not only the symptoms, (overeating, lack of motivation to exercise), but also the underlying root cause. "What do you want?" I asked her, and Tamara gave me the same answer every single one of the many clients I would have the privilege to work with were to give me: "To be happy". "What exactly is happiness to you? How do you think you will feel when you are happy, and what do you need to be, do, or have in order to feel those feelings?" I asked. Tamara was sure that her overeating was directly related to her body image. She was quite capable of "being good" on those days when she felt pretty, or when she was able to control her nutrition. But the moment something went wrong, she would head straight to the fridge for a "therapy" session with a good ice-cream.

Tamara had a history of anorexia. Back when she was admitted to a therapy center, she weighed 42 kilograms on 1.65. So food issues and body image were related from childhood, from as long as she could remember. Low self-esteem during adolescence predicts negative real-world consequences during adulthood (Trzesniewski, 2006). "Do you think you will feel better about yourself if you lose weight?" I asked. "This is highly unlikely unless you work on yourself from the inside. Nobody can give you approval except you. And that won't happen just because you drop a few kilos. Assuming you do finally get down to your goal weight, if you have low self-esteem you will almost surely find something else about yourself to dislike".

Anorexia nervosa: Tamara's past

Anorexia nervosa is an eating disorder characterized by immoderate food restriction and irrational fear of gaining weight, as well as a distorted body self-perception. It typically involves excessive weight loss (Hockenbury, 2008). Because of the fear of gaining weight, people with this disorder restrict the amount of food they consume. This restriction of food intake causes metabolic and hormonal disorders (Nogal, 2008). Anorexia nervosa is characterized by low body weight, inappropriate eating habits, obsession with having a thin figure, and the fear of gaining weight. It is often coupled with a distorted self-image, which alters how the affected individual evaluates and thinks about her or his body, food, and eating. (Rosen, 1995). The average caloric intake of a person with anorexia nervosa is 600–800 calories per day, (Tamara ate even less than that), and extreme cases of complete self-starvation are known. It is a serious mental illness with a high incidence of comorbidity and similarly high mortality rates of serious psychiatric disorders (Attia, 2010). Eating disorders in general and anorexia nervosa in particular have the highest mortality rate of any psychiatric disorder (Sullivan, 1995). Eating disorders are the result of a complex interplay of socio-cultural, familial, individual, and biological factors (Mizes and Bonifazi, 2001).

Body image disturbances are central to anorexia nervosa. At Utrecht University researchers found that at patients with anorexia nervosa and high levels of body dissatisfaction were related to more severe inaccuracies in the visual mental image of the body and overestimation of tactile distances. The results imply that body image disturbances not only affect visual mental imagery, but also extend to disturbances in somatosensory aspects of body image (Keizer, 2011).

Dr. Phil, maybe the most famous psychologist in America, conducted a series of television episodes about anorexia, aiming to make the problem more visual to the viewers who could not understand what went inside a patient's mind. He called for seven women to stand in a straight line, from the thinnest to the heaviest of all. He then asked the anorectic skeletal women to go and stand near the women she thinks share the same dimensions that she does. To the public's astonishment she took her place next to the two fattest ladies in the row.

Tamara's self-image and "inner picture" was similarly distorted during her "teen" years. Her parents sent her to recover from anorexia at the Shahaf Medical facility for eating disorders, located at the time in Kibbutz Naan in Israel. Shahaf provides treatment and prevention programs, an information and support center, and is committed to the advancement of research in this field. The treatment team includes a psychiatrist, clinical psychologists, family therapists, clinical dietitians, art therapists, and a drama therapist. The narrative approach focuses on separating the person and the problem, through the use of externalizing language. Treatment emphasizes a change in the patient's beliefs about their life, identity, and relationships. Different actions accrue when patients experience different relationships and perceive themselves as having new options. Eating disorders do not represent a person's bad intentions nor are they a manifestation of the pathological self. They are assumed to be the product of a disease that takes over a person's life and relationships. The approach focuses on recognizing the dominance of the disease and creating a coalition with the patient to fight it. One of the therapeutic techniques Tamara encountered there was indeed the mirror exposure in order to enable perspective and distance from the self. The goal of mirror exposure is one of decreasing judgment, neutralization, and acceptance not necessarily of positive evaluation of the body (Stewart, 2004). The team has helped many victims in their struggle to separate from their eating disorders, Tamara was one of them. The treatment at Shahaf enabled her to cope with her disorders within the community, and eventually make a complete recovery.

I met Tamara 6 years after her full recovery, back in California, almost 10 years ago. Physically Tamara was perfectly healthy. Weight-wise, she was overweight, (86 kilograms, 165 cm), and her body image, though 6 years have gone by after a full recovery from anorexia, was problematic. Tamara did not like her body, she still felt that her happiness depended on her being thin. Tamara kept old pictures of her weighing 58 kilograms, and this was her goal: Being once again a healthy, beautiful, thin girl, just like that girl in those pictures.

Tamara's nutrition plan

Tamar's weight loss was a huge challenge. Her body, after experiencing long months of fasting, was exhausted even though six years had passed. This was well reflected on the scale week after week. The pace of her weight-loss was so slow that Tamara was often on the verge of giving up. She did not. We trained three times a week, "according to the book": aerobic sessions, anaerobic sessions, intervals, cycle training and so forth. But the real challenge was the food. We needed Tamara to enjoy her meals. We needed her to avoid "starvation" and to fill her body with love in every bite she took. A healthy diet was in order, but there was room for a "fun dish" every week, of an additional 600 calories over which Tamara would fantasize. The "fun dish" was important psychologically: Delayed gratifications, an "award" for her hard work, awareness and preplanning;. Physiologically: An extra "unhealthy" 600 calories helped Tamara's body to avoid the famous plateau and to "awaken" her body from this "Metabolic Blackout".

Eventually Tamara's weight-loss was very slow, but she enjoyed the Gymind road she was on.

Foundation of Gymind: A WOW Moment

Tamar's story had a tremendous effect on the Gymind process. It was one day, after a long training session, when Tamara had already shed 10 percent of her body weight that she confided in me that her weight loss represented a huge "load off" of her chest. That those 400 calories the Polar watch showed she had burned represented 400 kilograms taken off of her soul, heart, and mind. That when she looked in the mirror, she no longer saw this unloved fat girl but an empowered young woman with wonderful abilities, strength, and a brighter future ahead of her. It was a wow moment for Tamara who decided to leave her boyfriend who "took her for granted" and "treated her with no respect", as she had been complaining during our sessions. It was not easy for her, but for her mental health it was a Must (The most amazing thing happened 4 months after their painful separation, when her boyfriend asked her to marry him, and indeed they were married the following year). I then clearly realized how body and mind are inseparable. I understood in a flash of insight, like a light bulb went on over my head, that work-out, nutrition and a profound "work-in" all three form the key to Tamara's happiness and THE foundation for the Gymind path. This WOW moment enabled Tamara and me to dig deeper and clean all "limiting beliefs" she had been keeping inside about herself, mainly about her body image. "I am only worth something when I am thin"; "I am only loved when I am thin"; Being skinny is the key to my happiness". The third chapter will discuss this issue thoroughly. But for now, fitness and nutrition were the keys which opened the door to release some old demons trapped inside Tamara's head and body for so many years and allowed her to see herself in a different light.

Psycho-Cybernetic Mechanism: How do you see yourself? How does your brain see yourself?

Maxwell Maltz wrote *Psycho-cybernetics* (1960), a system of ideas that he claimed could improve one's self-image. Maltz was a plastic surgeon. His life centered around giving people a good image of themselves when they looked in the mirror. As distinguished as he was in his field, he was at a loss to explain why a minority of patients were no happier after plastic surgery than before, even if disfiguring scars or other malformations had been removed. He found himself drawn to the new self-image psychology, which held that we generally conform in action and thought to a deep image of ourselves. Without a change to this inner image, patients would still feel themselves to be ugly, however excellent the cosmetic work. The book introduced Maltz's views, that a person must have an accurate and positive view of himself before setting goals, otherwise he will get stuck in a continuing pattern of limiting beliefs. His ideas focus on visualizing one's goals, and he believes that self-image is the cornerstone of all the changes that take place in a person. According to Maltz, if one's self-image is unhealthy or faulty, all of his efforts will end in failure (www.butler-bowdon.com).

Cybernetics is a word for how a system works and refers to the control-and-response systems found in some machines and animals, such as a thermostat or a missile guidance system. Let's say we're on a deep sea fishing trip, and I point the boat due north. You come up to me and say, "Hey, Joe, we're not catching any fish. Do you mind if we go somewhere else?" I say "Sure" and turn the wheel fifteen degrees. The boat starts to turn in a different direction, then suddenly shifts right back again, heading north like it was before. I turn the steering wheel forty degrees this time, so you can clearly see that the boat is going in a different direction. Just like before, the boat shifts back and heads north again. Now you're starting to get irritated., so I say, "I'll try even harder than I did before". I spin the wheel all the way around and turn the boat in the opposite direction. The boat starts to make a shift, then turns itself north yet again. Why does this keep happening? Because there's a cybernetic mechanism in this boat. Every time the boat deviates from its preprogrammed course, the cybernetic mechanism sends a signal to the automatic response mechanism to get the boat back onto its programmed course. In the same way, our brain has a cybernetic mechanism. Because of this mechanism, people win lotteries and then spend all the money, or they leave one abusive relationship and jump right into another one, or they lose weight and then gain it all back. Why? Because their thermostat is set at a certain level.

Your expectation points are already set, based on all of your past conditioning.

Unless you rewire the program, you'll revert right back to where you were before. Using will power and persistence alone will not work. This is where neuroplasticity really works well. We have to take the old brain - the old thermostat - and rewire it. We have to reset our thermostat before we can start seeing and behaving differently.

Exercising, eating right, and thinking right but also "changing the thermostat" is the only way for Tamara's long lasting success.

Affirmations: Set your goal

Repetitive affirmations such as "I want to lose weight", "I want to be thin", "I want to be healthy" might be similar to that Sisyphean spin of the wheel. First of all, your subconscious mind holds on to that "wanting" and constantly stays unsatisfied. Second of all, the work is superficial, linguistic, and "flat". If we rephrase the affirmation and get rid of the "wanting" and focus on the "having", that sets the mind in the right direction, and help us get in touch with our goal. Tamara gave up her "wanting to be thin" and began to "see" herself as a thin young lady: "Feel how you feel once you are there, have that picture in your mind and live that moment. That moment when your favorite pair of jeans finally fits. Hear yourself been complimented for your new figure."   For 21 consecutive days, Tamara wrote that affirmation:

"I want to weigh __58_____ kilograms

I am able to weigh _58_____ kilograms

I feel great when I weigh __58_____ kilograms

I weigh ____58_____ kilograms

Notice that those affirmations are in the present time and positively rephrased. The subconscious mind "lives" in the present and it does not "hear" the word "no". For example: The order "don't think of a blue tree" sets your mind directly into thinking about and even seeing that blue tree even though you were told not to.

Mindfulness and self-image

Mindfulness is "the process of drawing novel distinctions" or observing alternative perspectives through self-observation. (Langer, 2000). It is the moment-to moment perception of phenomena and the allowance of it to register with full awareness without the influence of cognitive shortcuts or distortions, desire, or expectations. This way of "being" sustains individuals in the present moment, allowing them to experience an awareness of their present situation. (Stewart, 2004). Mindfulness may be distinguished from constructs such as self-awareness by its nature of combining enhanced present moment awareness and a stance of nonjudgmentalism, neutrality, and acceptance of all experience. The "state" of Mindfulness includes a "wakefulness" and being in the moment that engages the "whole" individual, (body, mind and spirit), in the creation of our reality. Mindfulness is the way of being that allows individuals to develop new kinds of control, acceptances and compassion for the self in each moment. Mindfulness is the way to arrive at liberation from narrow views and obtain fearlessness and compassion (Hanh, 1975).

The 21-day guided imagination technique

The possibility of using the mind to free the self from ignorance, negativity, and delusion is the key to the development of compassion toward all things, including the Self. (Das, 1997). Mindful meditation, such as the 21 technique, seeks to enhance active engagement of the mind in the present moment, acknowledging experience (Stewart, 2004).

Body image is the picture that we have of what we look like in our heads. A body image ideal is how we wish we looked (Varnado-Sullivan, 2004).

When she suffered from anorexia nervosa, Tamara's picture in her head was very different from the one that the mirror actually showed her. In her mind she looked like she weighted over 80 kilograms, when in fact her weight dropped to 42 kg when admitted at the Shahaf Institute. The amazing thing was that when Tamara was cured, her weight went up to more than 80 kg, to the same image she had always possessed in her head.

A daily practice for at least 21 days of this imagination script a la NLP will help make an adjustment between the inner picture and the one reflected in the mirror. This visualization technique may eventually improve self-esteem and create a better and more "balanced" self-image. The prime message is: The responsibility of the shift is ours, and it is "imaginable" (in the sense of possible). The 21-day guided imagination technique is one of the ways to program our mind to see us in a positive way and make us feel loved, wanted, and complete. We thus form a "gestalt", a "model" or a "structure" into which we can melt down and remold positive behaviors and improved ways of thinking.

Stand up, reach out one hand in front of your body, palm facing up. Close your eyes and take three deep breaths. Imagine negativity, insecurity, doubts that are in your body flowing out of it and into your palm. Take it all out, don't leave anything inside. How does your palm feel like? What color does it have now?

Shake your hand or wash it with water.

Go back to standing up, closing your eyes, taking three deep breaths. Imagine a loved-one (your mother, your daughter, your brother) standing in front of you, looking at you with admiration and love. Take all that love and admiration and fill it inside those parts in your body that have been emptied of negativity, insecurity, doubts. There is now love there instead. What color does it have now?

Open your eyes to a "break state".

Close your eyes and take three deep breaths. Imagine yourself standing one step ahead of you. See yourself "painted" with the colors of that love and admiration you absorbed from your loved one. Look at yourself and notice how enlightened you look, secure, happy. Take one step forward into the "new you" and "lock" yourself inside.

Losing weight after 40: Mission impossible?

Starting in our early 40s, our bodies go through a series of changes that profoundly affect digestion, metabolism, and other bodily functions. Thanks to hormonal and other changes, the very growth rate of our cells slows down. It makes it even harder to lose extra fat (Haiken, 2013). Towards the age of 40, and with every year that goes by, many of my clients realize that the needle on the scale is a little harder to budge. What once used to really work (fasting for a day, over-exercising, avoiding chocolate for three days in order to lose those extra kilograms) is no longer working. You say "no thanks" to desert, you sign up for a Zumba class, and yet your jeans size goes up and your energy level goes down. The reasons? We have encountered many:

Thyroid problems strike as many as 1 out of 5 adults over age 40, most of them women. The most common of these is hypothyroidism - an underactive thyroid - and it's one of the primary reasons many women over 40 can't lose weight (American Thyroid Association, 2012). The thyroid is a gland that produces hormones that regulate metabolism, and when it's underactive, so is everything else. Symptoms include feeling cold all the time, poor circulation in the hands and feet, clammy hands, tiredness and lethargy, hair loss (including eyebrows and eyelashes) and weight gain, despite real attempts to exercise and eat well (Reinehr, 2002). Since 2003, the

American Association of Clinical Endocrinologists (AACE) has been recommending that a TSH test result of 2.5 or above should be considered a possible indicator of hypothyroidism. Many laboratories still use an older standard, according to which 5.5 is the cutoff above which TSH is considered abnormal. And new recommendations issued jointly by a task force of the AACE and the American Thyroid Association (ATA) didn't clarify things much; they basically say that a thyroid result of between 2.5 and 10 could indicate hypothyroidism on a case-by-case basis.

Sleep gets ever more elusive as you age. It's not just that we're busier and more stressed. We also have multiple physical issues, from back pain to snoring to night sweats, any of which can interfere with getting a good night's sleep. Yet, paradoxically, getting a good night's sleep is one of the keys to losing weight. In recent years, significant research has shown that lack of sleep is directly connected to weight gain because of the actions of two hormones, leptin and ghrelin, that control hunger and satiety, or feeling full. One key study concluded: "Sleep duration may be an important regulator of body weight and metabolism." Here's how it works: When you're sleep-deprived, ghrelin levels increase at the same time that leptin levels decrease. The result is more craving and less feeling full. Add to that the fact that sleep-deprived people often crave "energy" foods, which tend to be sweet or salty, and you can see how small changes in your routine can add up to big weight gain (Taheri, 2004; Ruesten, 2012).

Losing weight after 40 may seem like a "mission impossible". In fact, it's just more difficult and requires some extra awareness and focusing on the goal.

Aida's weight-loss at 45

We remember this brave 45-year-old mother of three, who at the age of 19 suddenly found herself with a broken thigh and two excruciating operations ahead of her. Aida's dream at 45 was to be able to run. She adopted a solid, smart, and consistent running program and is currently "living " her dream. Running was not her only goal. Aida, who at the time we started working together weighed 72.5 kilograms on 165 cm, wished to lose some weight. Her lowest ideal weight as a grown-up was 67, never under. And over the last 2-3 years, she had gained those extra kilograms she could not take off.

Running did the trick, no doubt about it. Thanks to at least three runs per week of 15-20 minutes, Aida felt like a "real runner", a "true professional athlete" and most importantly – the fat started to melt down. It was that intensity, that extra effort, the higher pulse in each training session that contributed to her weight loss success.

It was also the fact the Aida became more active during the day. She began to move and walk more inside the walls of her office, she went to grab her lunch instead of waiting for her secretary to do so for her, she escorted her youngest daughter to school, on foot. The more active Aida was, regardless of her steady runs, the higher her BMR climbed each and every day.

Nutrition wise: Aida had never been "much of an eater". She had always enjoyed healthy foods and maintained small portions as far the amount of calories she had consumed. However, she had been trying to lose those extra kilograms with no success so far. A "fine tuning" was needed to achieve the goal to a weight below the number of 67, maybe reaching for the first time in her life 65 kilograms. Not because the number itself mattered, but because it would reflect her new sporty life-style, her ability to break through some boundaries, and even help her improve her running by being thinner. Our goal was to keep Aida feeling full without succumbing to the temptation to eat like she could at age 20. One strategy was to eat more frequently but to consume less at each sitting. (An added benefit of eating this way is that it's easier to keep blood sugar steady, so we don't have the peaks and valleys that contribute to fatigue). Aida eats five to six small meals a day, and does not go more than three hours without eating. She drinks 10 glasses of water, no dietetic drinks, and goes to bed early.

We decided to listen to her body as far as gluten is concerned. When Aida replaces pasta with brown rice and bread with rice crispers or when quinoa replaces couscous, Aida feels better, more energetic – and she loses weight. It was not so much the gluten sensitivity she might be suffering from, if any. It was more about setting some limits, some boundaries. It's easier for Aida to say "no" to a waffle than to say "no" to a chocolate bar containing the same amount of calories but remains gluten free.

During the week-ends, Aida is much more aware of what she eats; she frequently takes pictures of her meals and shares with me her nutrition plan when it's harder to keep track of exactly what and how many calories are consumed (eating out on week-ends, being invited over at friend's house, etc.).

Aida's ideal Nutrition plan

Breakfast: 2 rice crackers with 1 tbsp. of home-made humus spread

Morning Snack: A cup of plum juice or a cup of orange juice

Lunch: A large bowl of vegetable salad with tahini sauce and a bowl of lentil soup.

Afternoon Snack: 7 almonds, 5 California nuts, 2 Brazil nuts

Dinner: Broiled salmon over 1 cup of green beans and 6 tbsp. of brown rice; two pieces of dark chocolate 60 % cocoa content.

"Don't drink your calories" (Jillian Michaels "The biggest loser's trainer")

One of the most inspirational reality TV shows would, to my eyes, be "The Biggest Loser". I believe there is not one viewer who cannot or would not relate to the difficulties the participants deal with on an every-day basis when they try to embrace a healthy life-style while fighting bad fitness habits and food temptations. We all encouraged them, cried with them when assignments were too hard for them to handle, and we watched, thrilled with admiration, as they shed pound after pound on their way to freedom. Free of surplus weight, free of former identity, free of hiding from their beautiful spirit. Jillian and Bob, the participant's trainers, often give advice and helpful tips (mainly promoting this or that heath product) and every now and then they say something that really makes a difference. "Don't drink your calories" is one of those tips, simple yet genius. You like to eat so much, save all those calories your body needs for eating and leave drinking out of the picture.

This also includes protein shakes. They contain many calories and should be considered as an alternative healthy snack or a small meal. When your goal is to maintain a healthy life-style and be in good shape, consuming a protein shake every morning is one of the best things you can do to give your metabolism a boost, according to Dr. Oz (2011). Not only does it nourish the body, but it also allows you to begin losing weight. An effective approach to weight management is to increase dietary protein or change the ratio of carbohydrate to protein in the diet (Krieger, 2006). This Illinois study demonstrates that increasing the proportion of protein to carbohydrate in the diet of adult women has positive effects on body composition, blood lipids, glucose homeostasis, and satiety during weight loss. (Layman, 2003; Skov, 1999; Noakes, 2005).

Not all protein shakes are created equal. Get familiar with labels and look for low-carb and low-fat whey proteins with almost no sugar. Whey protein is the best option, as soy or milk-based proteins are inferior sources that don't boost your energy-burning capabilities in the same way. In any case, we refer to any shake consumption as a balanced meal and not as a refreshing drink.

The power of water

One very powerful Israeli song "We are the children of that winter of 1973" talks about the disappointment of those kids born during the

"Yom Kippur War" since their parents promised them that this war would be the last war ever. Yours truly was born in those times, to a reality of war. In those days many people viewed buying products such as SodaStream that are manufactured in the settlements as contributing to sustaining the illegal settlements. That is why a number of organizations, Meretz USA, Americans for Peace Now, and Jewish Voice for Peace, as well as the Presbyterian and Methodist churches, have endorsed a boycott of SodaStream and other products made in the settlements. I was very young then, yet up until these days, like an old caressing memory, I can still hear the thrilling voice of Abie Nathan in that slogan played in "Kol Ha Shalom", (an offshore radio station that served the Middle East for 20 years, anchored off the coast of Tel Aviv. The station broadcast almost continuously between May 1973 and November 1993): "Drink water, cool refreshing water". It may be thanks to a national memory that I know how much water is best for us. So say No to "drinking our calories" means in the Gymind way: Say Yes to "drinking only water". More and more research proves how wrong and dangerous it is to consume artificial sweeteners or any sugar containing sodas for that matter. Despite safety reports of the artificial sweetener aspartame, health-related concerns remain (Schernhammer, 2012). Daily diet soft drink consumption was associated with several vascular risk factors and with an increased risk for vascular events (Gardener, 2012). Consumption of diet soda was significantly associated with an increased risk for diabetes in Japanese men. Diet soda is not always effective at preventing type 2 diabetes even though it is a zero-calorie drink (Sakurai, 2013). Dietetic beverages may increase appetite and may drives us to crave food even more (Beridot-Therond, 1998; (Renwick, 1994). Intake of Cola may be associated with low bone mineral density in women (Tucker, 2006).

If everyone knows soda is toxic for them, why do millions of people still indulge? They do. Maybe it's the "forever thin" and "thin at all price" international ethos, maybe it's due to ignorance, maybe it's the Quantitative Argument a la Perelman (1974) claiming "if everyone drinks it, we cannot all be wrong". Soda is tasty, cheap, convenient, and available everywhere, and it may not contain calories at all when it's the diet version. No matter where we go, we're bound to see an advertisement for some type of a can or a bottle of sugary or dietetic satisfaction. There's a reason advertisements exist, and it's not for aesthetics: Our brain is constantly processing every minute detail of information that our senses even remotely capture. Whether we remember it or not, all of this information is stored in our brain. If a Pepsi-Max advertisement steps into our peripheral vision for even a moment, it seeps into the murky depths of our mind and the next time our friend even mentions the word "Pepsi" or "Diet" our synapses fire, a connection is made to the instantaneous glance of the Pepsi Max advertisement, and our mouth begins to water. Why does it water? Because we are addicted, because we think we cannot do without, because we tell ourselves that it must be healthy or at least safe for our body since it's out there in the stores and since it appears on TV.

Sharon, 52, underwent a kidney transplant years prior to our encounter. She tells this amazing story of how hours after the successful operation, the doctor entered her room and without raising his eyes from the chart asked: "Are you drinking enough"? Sharon answered with full pride and confidence: "Yes, doctor, see how many bottles my husband brought in. I drink constantly". She tells how her doctor raised his eyes from the chart and to his horror, saw her drinking bottles of apple juice, orange juice, and sodas. Sharon now tells with a timid smile on her face how the doctor made her husband pour those bottles one by one into the toilet, ordering him to bring Sharon only water from that moment on. Sharon, who has been enjoying her new kidney for almost a decade, now drinks nothing but water.

How to quit that bad habit?

Whenever you are thirsty, your body will prefer water over any other drink. So indulge yourself with a cup of water and only then if you still feel the need, take a cup of soda.

Avoid bringing soda drinks into your home. Just like with food temptations: "Don't invite the enemy into your house".

Mix your favorite toxic soda with water, and each time add more and more water. Help your palate get used to a less sweet, healthier flavor.

Use the "like-to-dislike" NLP technique

Beth was 32 when her husband begged me to make her quit drinking diet cokes. "I carry those six packs every day and bring them home. Beth drinks them constantly. Not only is it expensive and heavy to carry, but Beth, who wants to lose weight, seems to be bigger than ever. Diet drinks don't seem to help her lose the extra weight. I love her dearly and I hate to see her suffering". Beth, who listened with teary eyes, gave me a firm look and said: "I wish I could quit this awful habit". We performed the "like to dislike" NLP technique. Beth hates grape juice. So her "dislike picture" was a tall glass filled with tasteless yucky grape juice that made her feel bad even just thinking about it. We switched the diet coke picture with that grape juice picture. It's been three years since then, and Beth is diet coke free, to both her and her husband's satisfaction.

How much water to consume?

Abie Nathan gave us a lot to think about concerning our national and social identity in his "Voice of Peace". We have suffered many more wars since that October war and unfortunately wars in the Middle-East may continue to take place. But for now we can begin by creating an inner peace and quiet in our body by simply choosing to drink water, cool refreshing water. How much of it? According to the Mayo Clinic staff (2011), this is a question with no easy answers. Studies have produced varying recommendations over the years, but in truth, your water needs depend on many factors, including your health, how active you are, and where you live (Sawka, 2005). Although no single formula fits everyone, knowing more about your body's need for fluids will help you estimate how much water to drink every day. Water is your body's principal chemical component and makes up about 60 percent of your body weight. Every system in your body depends on water. For example, water flushes toxins out of vital organs, carries nutrients to your cells, and provides a moist environment for ear, nose, and throat tissues. Lack of water can lead to dehydration, a condition that occurs when you don't have enough water in your body to carry out normal functions. Even mild dehydration can drain your energy and make you tired.

Every day we lose water through breathing, perspiration, and urine and bowel movements. For the body to function properly, we must replenish its water supply by consuming beverages and foods that contain water. So how much fluid does the average, healthy adult living in a temperate climate need? The Institute of Medicine determined (2011) that an adequate intake for men is roughly 3 liters (about 13 cups) of total beverages a day. The adequate intake for women is 2.2 liters (about 9 cups) of total beverages a day.

Aida has difficulties in consuming that amount of water each day. What does she do?

Aida puts reminders in her cell phone to drink every two hours.

You can ask a friend to remind you. Aida is receiving SMS and WhatsApp reminders from me.

Aida drinks a cup of water each time she eats something. 6 meals a day means 6 cups of water, and she is almost there.

Aida takes a bottle of water with her and puts it in front of her on her office desk.

Aida holds two bottles of water each time she goes for a run or a walk. Not only does she enjoy her water but she also trains with 2 weights of half a kilo.

What about caffeine intake?

Athletes are among the groups of people who are most interested in the effects of caffeine on endurance and exercise capacity (Burke, 2008). Caffeine is a common substance in the diets of most athletes, and it appears in many products, including energy drinks, sport gels, alcoholic beverages, and diet aids. It can be a powerful ergogenic [intended to enhance physical performance] aid at levels that are considerably lower than the acceptable limit of the International Olympic Committee and could be beneficial in training and in competition (Graham, 2001). Although many studies have investigated the effect of caffeine ingestion on exercise, not all are adequate to draw conclusions regarding caffeine and sports performance (Burke, 2008). Caffeine does not improve maximal oxygen capacity directly, but could permit the athlete to train at a greater power output and/or to train longer. It has also been shown to increase speed and/or power output in simulated race conditions. These effects have been found in activities that last as little as 60 seconds or as long as 2 hours (Graham, 2001). Caffeine's ability to enhance muscular work has been apparent since the early 1900s. However, the efficacy of caffeine ingestion for short-term high-intensity exercise is vague. A review of the literature revealed 29 studies that measured alterations in short-term performance after caffeine ingestion. Each study was critically analyzed using the Physiotherapy Evidence Database scale. Eleven of 17 studies revealed significant improvements in team sports exercise and power-based sports with caffeine ingestion, yet these effects were more common in elite athletes who do not regularly ingest caffeine. Six of 11 studies revealed significant benefits of caffeine for resistance training. Some studies show decreased performance with caffeine consumption when repeated sessions are completed. The exact mechanism explaining the ergogenic effect of caffeine for short-term exercise is unknown (Astorino, 2010). Further studies are needed to better elucidate the range of protocols (timing and amount of doses) that produce benefits and the range of sports to which caffeine may contribute (Burke, 2008).

And for the average active person, meaning us?

Caffeine is probably the most frequently consumed pharmacologically active substance in the world. It is found in common beverages, (coffee, tea, soft drinks), in products containing cocoa or chocolate, and in medications. Because of its wide consumption at different levels by most segments of the population, the public and the scientific community have expressed interest in the potential for caffeine to produce adverse effects on human health (Nawrot, 2003). People wake up each morning to the smell of hot coffee brewing, a tasty bitter-sweet way to kick-start the day. Many people drink coffee in the hope that it will aid their weight-loss efforts. While some research suggests it might (Westerterp-Plantenga, 2005; (Dulloo, 1999), experts differ greatly on whether coffee is a dieter's friend or foe. Drinking coffee might make you edgy, restless, and anxious. In fact, some studies speculate that coffee contributes to weight gain simply because you might eat more when you are nervous. On the MayoClinic website, dietician Katherine Zeratsky cautions against using coffee in your long-term weight loss plan. "Keep in mind that caffeine's a stimulant and too much can cause nervousness, insomnia, and other problems. Also, some caffeinated beverages, such as specialty coffees, are high in calories and fat. So instead of losing weight, you might actually gain weight." A modest and inverse relation to weight gain was discussed in a study by the Department of Health and Nutrition Sciences, Brooklyn College. The researchers suggest that drinking coffee may actually result in decreased weight. Since the improvement was modest, the study cautioned against consuming coffee as a weight-loss aid. Coffee also may raise blood pressure, the study found, stating "Caffeine and caffeinated coffee have been shown to acutely increase blood pressure and thereby to pose a health threat to persons with cardiovascular disease risk" (Greenberg, 2006).

According to scientists at the University of Georgia, drinking about a cup of coffee before you start exercising limits muscle pain when working out. With less pain during your workout, you may exercise longer and more frequently, increasing the calories your body burns (Motl, 2003). Another study found that caffeine consumed one hour prior to exercise can improve endurance exercise performance (Hodgson, 2013).

Because coffee is a stimulant, drinking too much of it may keep you awake at night, compromising your seven to nine hours of restful sleep. Research by scientists at the University of Chicago shows a correlation between lack of sleep and weight gain (Nedeltcheva, 2010).

High caffeine consumption has been proposed as a risk factor for osteoporotic fracture, but the evidence associating high caffeine intake with low bone density is inconsistent. However, a Mayo Clinic study found that among elderly women, in whom calcium balance performance is impaired, high caffeine intake may predispose to cortical bone loss from the proximal femur (Cooper, 1992).

It is known now that consumption of moderate amounts of caffeine is even beneficial for these goals:

Increases energy availability

Increases daily energy expenditure

Decreases fatigue

Decreases the sense of effort associated with physical activity

Enhances physical performance

Enhances motor performance

Enhances cognitive performance

Increases alertness, wakefulness, and feelings of "energy"

Decreases mental fatigue

Quickens reactions

Increases the accuracy of reactions

Increases the ability to concentrate and focus attention

Enhances short-term memory

Increases the ability to solve problems requiring reasoning

Increases the ability to make correct decisions

Enhances cognitive functioning capabilities and neuromuscular coordination (Glade, 2010).

Meet Charlene and her addiction to caffeine

When Charlene, 29, a single mother of 2, and a smoker, came to me a year ago with 10 extra kilograms, it was probably the caffeine intake that caught my attention more than anything else. Charlene consumed more than 10 cups of coffee each day, on a relatively "normal" day. On some more hectic days maybe even more than that. Cigarettes and coffee apparently go together, so the more she smoked, the more cups of coffee she drank. It's that simple. Since one of the first steps that Gymind believes in is "drink water, cool refreshing water" Charlene was asked to reduce her caffeine intake to the maximum recommended amount which is 3 cups a day. My advice to her was also to control the amount of caffeine powder she puts in a cup. A "flat" tsp. is enough. Charlene made the change. She increased her water intake to 10 cups of water a day and only 3 "weak" cups of coffee. She suffered from severe headaches for three days, knowing it was a true reaction of her body cleansing itself from caffeine. Charlene has been smoking less since then. She had been losing weight so quickly, as if her body cleansed itself from caffeine and from all the rest: nicotine, fats, and bad habits.

Alcohol intake for your health

It sounds like a mixed message: Drinking alcohol may offer some health benefits, especially for your heart. On the other hand, alcohol may increase your risk of health problems and damage your heart. According to the Mayo Clinic Stuff (2011), when it comes to drinking alcohol, the key is doing so only in moderation. Results from observational studies, where alcohol consumption can be linked directly to an individual's risk of coronary heart disease, provide strong evidence that all alcoholic drinks are linked with lower risk (Rimm, 1996). The latest dietary guidelines make it clear that no one should begin drinking or drink more frequently on the basis of potential health benefits. So don't feel pressured to drink alcohol. But if you do drink alcohol and you're healthy, there's probably no need to stop as long as you drink responsibly and in moderation.

Health benefits of moderate alcohol use:

Reduce your risk of developing heart disease

Reduce your risk of dying of a heart attack

Possibly reduce your risk of strokes, particularly ischemic strokes

Lower your risk of gallstones

Possibly reduce your risk of diabetes

Moderate alcohol use may be of most benefit only if you're an older adult or if you have existing risk factors for heart disease, such as high cholesterol (Mukamal, 2006). If you're a middle-aged or younger adult, some evidence shows that even moderate alcohol use may cause more harm than good (Quintana, 2013). In fact, if you're a woman and drink alcohol, talk to your doctor about taking supplemental folate to help reduce the risk of breast cancer associated with alcohol use (Coronado, 2011). Drinking low to moderate amounts of alcohol may delay age-associated cognitive decline in older women, including slowing deterioration in global cognitive function (Stott, 2008).

The 2010 Dietary Guidelines for Americans recommend that if you choose to drink alcohol, you do so only in moderation, up to one drink a day for women or two drinks a day for men.

Examples of one drink include:

Beer: 355 milliliters

Wine: 148 milliliters

Distilled spirits: 44 milliliters

Bethany, a 22 young lady, followed her cousin Muriel (whom we have already met) in order to lose some weight (40 kilograms, which she did shed over the course of three years) and maintains a healthy life style. Apparently, besides over-eating (mostly carbs and sweets) she had the habit of drinking a lot, mostly with friends at bars and discothèques. Beer was her favorite drink. 6 months prior to our encounter, she had gained more than 10 kilograms just by increasing her alcohol intake. The first week in the Gymind process, she lost 3.2 kilograms thanks to drinking only water and eating smart.

You should avoid the use of alcohol when:

- You're pregnant or trying to become pregnant.

- You take medications that can interact with alcohol.

- You've had a previous hemorrhagic stroke.

- You've been diagnosed with alcoholism or alcohol abuse.

- You have liver or pancreatic disease.

- You have heart failure or you've been told you have a weak heart or dilated cardiomyopathy.

- You're planning to drive a vehicle or operate machinery.

Not the end: Know yourself, set a goal, and choose a nutrition plan that fits your needs

Skinny-fat Ili, Aida the runner, Matt the pediatrician, Tamara the former anorectic girl, Hanna the future dentist, Muriel and her cousin Bethany, kids like Oliver, Tami, and Liana (and their families) - they are all seeking a way for happiness and well-being. It's in this chapter that we followed their search for better nutrition and better diet. Knowledge gives them power. The power to know how to treat their body better, how to feed it properly and when. It's with that power that they can look in the mirror and accept what they see, even love their reflection. They are all in a place where they communicate better with themselves. Knowing what they love to eat, what foods are better for them. They are now more powerful, thanks to that. That knowledge of what to eat and when to eat it gives them the power to better interact with their body and mind and to empower themselves even more from the inside-out. Embracing the right diet-for-you is not a "moment to moment" decision. It's a road you walk through day after day, moment to moment. Your goal does not necessarily wait for you at the end of the road. ("Thank god I reached 58 kilograms, now I can eat whatever, whenever"). The road is the goal itself. You then act every day AS IF you weigh 58 kilograms even if you are not there yet. Knowing yourself is important: your BMR levels, your weight, your body fat percentage, what you love to eat, for example. But also know yourself as far as what you need to eat in order to feel good and look good. Set a goal. Whether it's to lose weight, stay healthy, lose fat for more muscle tissue or better educate your children about eating smart and good nutrition. Eat smart, drink water, listen to your culinary needs, and consume them with moderation. Enjoy every bite and allow yourself the indulgence in temptation every now and then. You will regain control over your life, feeling empowered and accomplished. Preplanning your meals and having an awareness of what you need and desire are the key for that holistic feeling and one of the crucial components along with fitness and soul searching for a healthy, happy, best – You.

Chapter III

The power of the mind, therapy, and change

Primary thought: The power of your mind on your body

Physical activity and smart nutrition are only one part of the equation for a complete and healthy life-style. Complement the third part in the equation for our health: The power of the mind and the ability of the brain: Our thoughts, our emotions, our words and our dreams, hence our Mind. As a trainer I have experienced many "breakthrough" sessions over the years, personally and professionally, having the privilege to escort people along their journey, becoming a true believer in Gymind as a way of life, as a "treasure chest" providing many wonderful tools for life. This third chapter deals with the power of the subconscious mind as a critical part of the Gymind way for good health.

Our essence holds tremendous power over our life and may and will influence our body. If the other two chapters deal with the impact of the Doing over the Being in the sense of "we exercise to feel better" or "we eat smart for good health", this current chapter takes us higher into the brain, into the spiritual side of our existence and deeper into our heart and emotions, allowing us to touch the unattainable, to dialogue sometimes with what might be unseen or unheard and to explore the endless opportunities that lie in our mind: Unlimited emotions and thoughts inside the limits of our skull.

The mind may be intangible, sometimes elusive, but it's a part of who we are, it defines who we are and it must be explored. How we relate to our brain affects every cell in our body. Our thoughts and feelings are part of numerous feedback loops that influence every tissue and organ. So we explore that feedback, that connection between our

Mind and our Body. One of the fundamental rules in the NLP theory we are about to encounter could not conclude better, than by stating that "Mind and body are parts of the same system" (Faulkner, 1991).

We are living in a golden age of brain research. New breakthroughs emerge constantly, revealing the astonishing power of the brain to heal, create, and evolve. Aging is associated with progressive losses in function across multiple systems, including sensation, cognition, memory, motor control, and affect. The traditional view has been that functional decline in aging is unavoidable because it is a direct consequence of brain machinery wearing down over time. In recent years an alternative perspective has emerged (Mahncke, 2006). Where scientists once believed that the brain's hardwiring couldn't be changed, we now know that the brain is constantly evolving and our ability to rewire our brains remains intact from birth to the end of life. Researchers have also dispelled the myth that aging in the brain and memory loss are inevitable and irreversible. No matter how old we are, our brain is incredibly resilient and has the capacity to create new neural pathways if we choose to keep learning and opening ourselves to new experiences (Chopra, 2012).

This is the present study's basic assumption and axiomatic point of view: Our brain can evolve and change, new cells are born; new neurological paths are made, cemented into the existing neural networks if they are challenged by a novel learning experience, by novel sets of behaviors. We have the control and maybe even the responsibility to make our brain, hence our body, react and develop. Tanzi and Chopra in their "Super Brain" book (2012) make a distinction between what they call the "baseline brain" and the super brain. The baseline brain is the everyday brain that runs unconsciously in the background to keep us alive and healthy. That's not a minor role; the baseline brain is a marvel of complexity and efficiency. But too much of it is devoted to habit, old conditioning, and unconscious reflexes. We believe that the brain is designed to deliver much more. Through practices and techniques of self-awareness and conscious choice making, we can transform our baseline brain into a super brain (Tanzi, 2012). And it's up to us to decide, whether we are active or passive. Whether we continue to follow old habits and conditioning or create new and improved ones. We are not our brain. We are the user of our brain. Our brain looks to us for instructions, guidance, and inspiration. Let us charge and recharge it with goodness and positivity in order to feel good, positive, all over our body.

Be at cause: Because you take control

The belief that "anything is possible" forms the foundation of the Gymind method, as nurturing and enabling a healthy way of life. Certainly, we are born with specific DNA. According to Agus,(2012), who claims to speak on behalf of conventional medicine, DNA is "given" to us by our parents and we have no choice. In this regard DNA is practically accidental. Just as accidents happen so does DNA without our having much say in the matter". We have a certain appearance, whether we resemble our father or our mother; our brain is shaped in a certain way; we hold a very rich and profound set of beliefs and thoughts. We are unique, each and every one of us; we are different from one another and should be proud of that. Our life experience plays a vital role in shaping who we are now, and who we would grow up to be in the future. We are invited to believe that we can change our own experience, and that we can learn how to do it. But most of all, it means that we get some control over what happens in our brain. Most people are prisoners of their own brains (Bandler, 1985). It's as if they are chained to the last seat of the bus and someone else is driving. You should drive your own bus. If you don't give your brain a little direction, either it will just run randomly on its own, or other people will find ways to run it for you – and they may not always have your best interests in mind.

The first thing Michael Stevenson, founder of "Transform Destiny", taught in his seminar was that our duty as therapists was to show people they should always be on the side of the C, as far as possible from the side of the E. C equals Cause and E equals Effect. We should be "at cause", be Cause it all begins with us. Without blaming the Effect, the consequences, others. Phrases such as: "The floor is crooked that's why I cannot dance" or "The cake was just there so I had to eat it" mean being at the E side of the equation. Whereas "I need to improve my dance skills" of "I will take only this small piece of cake" means placing ourselves as close as we can to the C side of the equation.

Where are you located? This may be the first question I present to my clients.

$$C < E$$

As children we have egocentric thinking that predominates during this period of cognitive development (Dworkin, 1988), thinking that "we are the world" and that everything revolves and evolves around us. As babies we cover our eyes with our hands thinking nobody can see us, since we cannot see anything: "Where am I ? Peek-a-boo"... We are basically egocentric human beings. However, when we grow up, society teaches us to consider others, in the spirit of "give the bigger piece of cake to your friend". The implicit, or what the subconscious mind instantly understands by that, would be "he matters more than you". And for giving up on our egocentric behavior - we get rewarded: "very nice, you are a good friend and a polite host". Mixed signals? Oh yes. On one hand "we are the world", on the other "there is another world out there to consider, it may matter more than mine". And in time we might lose that connection to the inner voice, to that inner world, to that egocentric kid that was deprived over time from things he desired, from himself. In the previous chapter we discussed our need to go back to breathing right, through our belly, just like we used to as babies; or enjoying physical activities just like we used to enjoy it as care-free, active, and joyful kids. The C can also stand for "Child" and the E for "Everybody Else". Or C for "Choices" I Can Carry as opposed to E of "Everything Else". By pulling us back to the "C" side, Stevenson's intentions (2007) are to bring us back to those endless opportunities we are born with and may have naturally lost or forgot about along the way. To bring us back to "cause" without losing this connection to the outer world or better yet, make this a better connection, an improved one, summon abundance, positivity in life and good mental and physical health.

Irene is taking charge

We remember Irene, who at the age of 37 after giving birth to her third child, was diagnosed with Lupus. For the first several weeks Irene stayed in bad: Weak, feeble, dysfunctional. She used to wake up with stiff joints, mainly in her hands (a known symptom in Lupus syndrome) which made it even harder on her to perform her every-day chores as a wife and a mother. Most of all, her spirit was broken. Irene had two choices: Stay in bad all day feeling sorry for herself (with every justification to do so) or do something. When the system of support around her that consisted of her husband and her mother gently urged her to DO something to improve her situation, Irene decided to fight back against Lupus. She decided to take charge, to be "at cause". Years after that decision (which also made her come for Gymind sessions), she will have confided to me that an enlightening thought went through her mind one morning, while she rinsed and massaged her stiff fingers under the warm relaxing tap water. She thought that she still has the same body. The body that gave birth three times to three perfect boys, that enabled her to exist in good condition for 37 years. It's that same body that "summoned" Lupus into it for some reason. So it's that body that can fight it back and make the lupus disappear.

Emma is taking charge

In chapter two we fleetingly mentioned Emma, 55, who was tired of those diet trends, who had tried them all, who almost gave up on a great figure and better health. When she contacted me, Emma's condition was poor, in the sense that she almost did not believe in her ability to take charge. She had been sitting for so long in the back seat of the bus, allowing everybody else to hold the steering wheel. Emma needed to know herself first, to reconnect with her inner voice, to recharge herself emotionally and mentally in order to make a change. She is still in the process of doing so, but for the first time in her life, she realizes that this is the right way to go. Blaming other won't help; focusing on your own doing- definitely will.

Barak is taking charge

Barak, 28, the acupuncturist we met in Chapter One, took charge and got back into running in order to regain control over his life. He also had to make a decision about his spouse: Should he stay in that marriage or not. We remember how Barak felt his love life going down the hill without his having any control of it. Our main goal in his Gymind process was to make Barak focus on himself, not to point an accusing finger at his wife, or anyone else for that matter. Focus on what he can control, on what he can take charge of: His body, his career, his thoughts, his sets of beliefs, and his dreams.

Look at the mirror to spot flaws

It was when I was in my early 20s that my mother took me to some of those long "awareness" seminars. For almost a year, twice a week for an hour and a half, I was submerged in fascinating lectures about "new thinking" and "recreating your reality", long before we heard about "The Secret" by Rhonda Byrne (2006), and long before Robin Sharma excited millions of readers with "The Monk Who Sold his Ferrari" (1999). That maybe was the first time I encountered the ability to take charge over things you cannot really touch, over your thoughts that you could not control: Your mind. I remember specifically that brilliant metaphor that the professor presented for us:

"Let's say you have a spot of dirt on your nose. Either I tell you that you have it, or you go and look in the mirror to spot it. What do you do? Let's say you take a napkin and start wiping the dirt off the mirror. Since the dirt is seen there. So you wipe it off and you wipe it off really hard. Then what happens? You are getting tired, the muscles in your arms begin to cramp, you may get angry and frustrated because nothing helps, the dirt won't wipe off the mirror. You then decide to take the napkin and easily and gently pass it over your face, right where the dirt was spotted in the mirror. What happens now? When you now look in the mirror, the dirt is gone".

The world is a mirror for us. It's a wonderful tool to help us spot all those small irritating dirty spots we carry inside. Instead of blaming the outer world, pointing out what goes wrong there, (which may cause us frustrations, muscle cramps and anger), we simply take charge of our own cleaning, even thanking the world for pointing it out to us. Ceasing to blame "the world" and placing the focus on the self is the key element to attaining your goal according to Gymind. It's only after we take care of our personal development and growth, that we can see changes in "the world". Certainly, the world out there always helps us, through reciprocity, communication, and relationships to spot those flaws.

So life and 'mind' are systemic processes. The processes that take place within a human being and between human beings and their environment are systemic. Our bodies, our societies, and our universe form an ecology of complex systems and sub-systems, all of which interact with and mutually influence each other. It is not possible to completely isolate one part of the system from the rest of the system. Such systems are based on certain 'self-organizing' principles and naturally seek optimal states of balance or homeostasis (Dilts, 2011).

Irene took charge over her body. She began to exercise, hence strengthened her muscles and improved her cardio-vascular abilities.

She felt better after a good cardio work-out, thanks to endorphins and adrenalin she produced in her brain. Researchers at the University of Dublin in Ireland conducted a study on the cognitive effects of exercise, stating that exercise elevates levels of brain neurotrophic factor; proteins that have been the subject of many recent studies and are now known to promote the growth of healthy nerve and muscle cells, respectively. The emotional component is undeniable because exercise helped Irene so much with her bad moods and depression (Clark, 2011). Irene chose her nutrition better, by reading labels and making better choices on each meal she cooked for herself and her family. But far more than that, Irene started to speak differently and think differently. She shifted the point of view of her mind from being the victim, ("I am the target of Lupus"), from being deprived of her happiness, ("I feel so bad because I am a dysfunctional mom"), to being her own rescuer. She gained so much out of it, not just her physical health.

When Irene first came to me, her marriage was in jeopardy. She hated "the world" for putting her in misery and she saw everything in "black or white": "I am either sick or healthy, either happy or sad;, either my husband supports me or he does not". The Gymind method in general and NLP in particular had a lot to do with her recovery. From the victim she became the rescuer, from a martyr she was transformed into a redeemer (and started to help her friends in need, spreading love and happiness around her). Irene gradually transformed into a happy, positive person who fell in love once again with the husband she stopped constantly blaming and began to see the world as a place of endless opportunities and multiple colors. She found balance and stability in her life.

Fundamental rules of the subconscious mind

In order to create a profound and meaningful change in the way we think, live, and behave and to strive for better mental and physical health, it's essential to identify several ground rules of the subconscious mind.

The subconscious constantly "lives" in the present time. When we recall a memory and tell about it, we can see, hear and feel this event "as if it is happening now". We see that in our eyes, our breathing, and the way we talk about the event. At any given moment ALL the memories are stored subconsciously in our mind and our body. Think about it like the rings on the trunk of a tree. Each ring tells how old the tree is, yet the tree itself grows vertically and not horizontally and you cannot see the rings from the outside. In that sense the past is constantly within us, as if living in the present time, constantly accompanying our growth.

The subconscious mind works with simplicity and minimum efforts. It's "just there", we cannot argue with it. We breathe, we walk, we move our eyes, and we hear. Those are all biological mechanisms that operate subconsciously. Thoughts come to our mind "just like that", naturally. Katy Byron (2002) would say "thoughts are like the breeze or the leaves on the trees or the raindrops falling. They appear like that (…) would you argue with a raindrop?"

The subconscious mind cannot differentiate between reality and imagination, and it takes everything personally. When we dream we may have physiological reactions: Sweat, racing heartbeats, or a sense of fear. Dreams reside in our imagination, yet the subconscious reacts as if they were real. Almost the same thing happens with a movie that makes us feel good or when we hear a song and experience strong emotions. The subconscious mixes imagination and reality, but it also takes everything personally making us relate to the story-line of a movie or a book and create identification with the characters. This rule enables us to empower ourselves with words, even if we refer to others. When we complement a friend, the subconscious takes it personally, it's as if we complemented ourselves. The mind does not have eyes nor does it have ears. Our thoughts and words nourish the mind's perception of what is true. So we have to use them wisely.

The subconscious mind cannot process negative words like "no", "not" or "don't". If we are asked not to think about a blue tree, we are almost compelled to instantly think and maybe even see in our mind a blue tree. Affirmations and other forms of self-talk are more effective when phrased and presented positively. We should replace: "I will not eat from this cake today" with "I will eat an apple", or "I will only eat one piece of cake".

As a protective measure, the subconscious mind will repress memories of experiences that contain unresolved negative emotions. Although the memories are buried, the beliefs and emotions attached to them will continually affect a person's behavior and he is bound to meet them over and over again on many occasions to come. We can refer to this as an old phonograph and records. The record turns under the phonograph needle, but if there is even a tiny crumb on the record it will encounter this crumb on each and every round it takes, so that the music would get stuck on the same line over and over again. It is important to recognize all those "crumbs" in our life, release them and allow the music to play peacefully.

The subconscious mind cannot bear conflicts of any kind. It strives for harmony and inner peace. Internal conflicts occur when two or more "parts" of a person lead to behaviors which are contradictory. The most problematic conflicts occur when the opposing parts have negative judgments about each other. We are beset by conflicts when inner wishes collide with outside circumstances. We want to eat the cake and leave it whole; we want to have a thriving career yet be able to raise our kids properly and spend time with them. We want to lose weight yet need to have some more of that delicious ice-cream. A part of us wants to become healthier by exercising regularly while another part wants to enjoy relaxing in front of the television. Conflicts are there constantly. However, the right dialogue with the subconscious mind can help us create an " integration of parts " which helps resolve the conflict. A "magical" technique allows us to integrate parts at the unconscious level and to find a higher level of wholeness (Stevenson, 2007).

Hana: To eat the chocolate bar or not to eat it? That is the conflict

Hana, the 22 year old girl we met in Chapter 1, continues with her daily training sessions and keeps a fairly healthy life-style. One of our most significant sessions touched upon part of conflicts in Hana's life. She wishes to have a great career as a dentist, just like her father, yet she wants to be a "soccer-mom" just like her mother. Hana wants to become a dentist, yet considers herself very artistic and thinks about Art as a profession. Just like Hana we face many conflicts that our subconscious "suffers" from on a daily basis. As a result, Hana may become indecisive, incomplete and she may feel guilt and other negative emotions such as fear, anger, or sadness. With "Parts Integration" we take one conflict as a prototype, we create an integration, and call for all the other conflicts that lie somewhere in our subconscious to rejoin in the integration (Radwan, 2013). A wonderful magical "mind-body" technique we are about to explore with Hana:

In order to identify both parts of the conflict, hold both of your hands in front of you so that your palms face the ceiling. Look at the first hand and imagine that you are holding the first part of the conflict. Who\what do you see? (Hana saw herself sitting on that hand, but it can be anyone or anything). Do the same for the second part. (Again, Hana saw herself sitting on the other hand, representing the other part of the conflict).

Hana, please look at the first part and ask it "why do you want to eat that chocolate bar?"

Hana: "Because I want you to enjoy the taste of chocolate"

Again: "Why do you want me to enjoy the taste?"

Hana: "Because I want you to be happy".

Again: "Why do you want me to be happy"?

Hana: "Because I want you to feel alive"

We ask more and more questions until we determined the highest positive intention of the part: To be happy, alive, complete and healthy.

We then asked the second part about its intentions, using the same "chunking-up" method. Our main goal was allowing the two parts to agree on a common goal which was happiness or feeling alive, in Hana's case. The more we go up the hierarchy of intentions, the more we find that both parts are actually on the same page, together, supporting the same goal and each other.

We now talk to both parts and tell them that they both have the same intention and that there is no need for a conflict. We call for other parts that were also once part of the larger whole and we invite them to join the integration.

This is the magical part when Hana's hands are coming closer and closer until they touch. This sends a clear message to the subconscious mind that the conflict was resolved and that other conflicts have joined the integration. Hana takes both hands and puts them on her chest, as if taking the integrated parts inside and have them merge into the wholeness inside.

In the future, Hana won't find that great resistance when she tries to stop herself from eating chocolate.

NLP: Neuro Linguistic Programming and the key for change

NLP is a state-of-the-art set of communication methods for enhancing personal and professional development and for creating personal change gracefully (Faulkner, 1991). The neurological system regulates how our bodies function, language determines how we interface and communicate with other people, and our programming determines the kinds of models of the world we create. Neuro Linguistic Programming describes the fundamental dynamics between mind (neuro) and language (linguistic) and how their interplay affects our body and behavior (programming) (Dilts, 2011). NLP is also described as "the software of your brain" allowing you to automatically tap into the kind of experiences you want to have (Faulkner, 1991). As human beings we can never know reality, we can only know our perceptions of reality. We experience and respond to the world around us primarily through our sensory representational systems. It is our 'neuro-linguistic' maps of reality that determine how we behave and that give those behaviors meaning, not reality itself. It is generally not reality that limits us or empowers us, but rather our map of reality (Dilts, 2011). That map can be changed by studying the structure of subjective experience. By creating models of human excellence in which usefulness, not truthfulness, is the most important criterion for success, we reach our goal of this healthy transformation (Faulkner, 1991).

There is a powerful way to re-program our brain, a way to change our relationship with eating, sleep, sex ,and basic emotions like fear, love, and aggression (Becker, 2012). Humans share with animals a primitive neural system for processing emotions such as fear and anger. Unlike other animals, humans have the unique ability to control and modulate instinctive emotional reactions through intellectual processes such as reasoning, rationalizing, and labeling our experiences (Hariri, 2000). While cognitive therapies can modify behavior, they are of questionable help in altering these basic drives, since they may not go "deep" enough (Becker, 2012). Our drives are largely governed by two small primitive brain structures, the hypothalamus and the amygdala, the size of a pea and an almond respectively, representing less than 1% of the brain's 1.2 kilograms of neural matter. Together, they constitute the control center of the paleomammalian brain, the "limbic" brain, that governs our basic urges and desires as well as our homeostatic "set points" for temperature, sleep, body fat, and behavioral urges like sex drive and aggression (Joseph, 2012).

We can attempt to change your behavior by conscious determination and cognitive therapies. But most attempts at intentional change are temporary and are doomed to fail in the long term because they are strongly resisted by powerful homeostatic processes encoded in our limbic brain. Modern medicine recognizes the importance of homeostatic drives, and has developed pharmaceuticals to override them with diet pills, sleeping pills, and antidepressants. In fact, these medications do shift the balance of neurotransmitters and neural activity, at least in the short term. But such chemical interventions are short-sighted "crutches" that promote dependency and come with side effects. Often they exhibit a "tolerance" effect: The brain's control system fights back and weakens the impact of the medication. To maintain the benefit, doses are increased, but this strategy may not always work (Becker, 2012).

The anatomy of the brain at a glance

The figure below provides a "macro" view of the major parts of the limbic system. Located at the center of the brain, perched atop the brainstem, the limbic system includes not only the hypothalamus and amygdala, but other structures such as the hippocampus, cingulate gyrus, pituitary gland. (Gloor, 1997; MacLean, 1990). The amygdala is connected tightly by numerous nerve bundles to the hypothalamus. The amygdala acts directly on the hypothalamus to control hypothalamic drives and conversely, the hypothalamus "uses" the amygdala, (and to some extent the septum), as a window on the world to satisfy its drives by selectively searching out appropriate foods, potential mates, and sleep and exercise opportunities. (Markakis, 1997). The amygdala is particularly sensitive to sound with valence or meaning, such as vocalizations, crying, or music. The amygdala plays a central role in auditory fear conditioning, regulation of the acoustic startle response and can modulate auditory cortex plasticity. A stressful acoustic stimulus, such as noise, causes amygdala-mediated release of stress hormones, which may have negative effects on health, as well as on the central nervous system. On the other hand, short-term exposure to stress hormones elicits positive effects such as hearing protection. (Kraus, 2012).

Reaching the Amygdala and reprograming some of those "primitive" emotional and mental perspectives would be the key to a change.

We have already encountered some major NLP wonders: The Swish Pattern, in order to change a behavior and erase bad habits; the Like to Dislike technique in order to help us make better nutrition choices; The 21-day Technique that helps to change the inner picture and summon confidence and self-love. We have mentioned briefly the "mind games" at the gym and how "reprogramming that little voice inside your head" can push you to do and be better. In fact, many of us live and practice some of these tools intuitively without even knowing it's a method, a smart way to enhance a change and to make us grow as human beings. NLP is not just a field. It can be a way of life in many ways (Stevenson, 2004). Those "mind tools" support that cognitive and conscious determination to change and lead the brain to explore new neurologic pathways through a reprogramming of the amygdala.

Submodalities in NLP

We have already discussed how as humans we experience the world subjectively, thus, we create subjective representations of our experience. These subjective representations of experience are constituted in terms of five senses and language. That is to say, our subjective conscious experience is in terms of the traditional senses of vision, audition, tactition, olfaction and gustation such that when we, for example, rehearse an activity "in our heads", recall an event or anticipate the future we will "see" images, "hear" sounds, "taste" flavors, "feel" tactile sensations, "smell" odors and think in some (natural) language. (Grinder, 1976). Furthermore, these subjective representations of experience have an apparent structure, a pattern. It is in this sense that NLP is sometimes defined as the study of the structure of subjective experience (Dilt, 1980). Behavior can be described and understood in terms of these sense-based subjective representations which we refer to in NLP as Submodalities, those fine distinctions or the subsets of the Modalities ,(Visual, Auditory, Kinesthetic, Olfactory, Gustatory, and Audio digital), that are part of each representational system that encode and give meaning to our experiences. They are the building blocks of the representational systems by which we code, order, and give meaning to the experiences we have. Submodalities are how we structure our experiences. For example, in visual terms, common distinctions include: brightness, degree of color (saturation), size, distance, sharpness, focus, and so on; in auditory terms: loudness, pitch, tonal range, distance, clarity, timbre, and so on. (NLPWorld.co.uk).

Belle's encounter with NLP

We met Belle and her husband Leroy in a previous chapter, as the couple who adopted the pedometer as a tool to motivate them to be more active. They both strive to maintain a healthy life style, despite or thanks to Belle's heart condition and the operation she underwent as an infant. They both try to lose weight. Leroy has shed 10 kilograms, Belle five, so far. Since they embraced Gymind as a way of life more than three years ago, weight matters less and it's the road they take that matters most. One of the many sessions we have held over the years dealt with Belle's strong image of her father pointing a finger at her and telling her: "Belle, you have eaten enough, put your fork down". This image won't leave her and apparently it's a huge hurdle as far as losing the extra weight. Each time she takes a bite, her father's image reappears and so she wonders: Have I had enough to eat? Should I put my fork down? She often eats more than she needs out of spite. Even though she is no longer five years old, even though her dad is no longer near her, this memory still lives on in her mind, controls her way of thinking and her experience regarding foods and eating habits.

We had to "release" Belle from that image stored deep down in her mind.

Dissociation. Belle is looking at that little girl, (herself at the age of 5), dissociated.

She now observes the submodalities:

The image of that 5-year-old girl and the girl's dad: This image, is it bright or dim? Colored or black and white? How much color? Is it big or small? Is it near or far? In focus or out of focus?

The sound of the dad's voice: Is it loud or soft? Is it high pitched or low pitched? Does it have a range? Is it near or far? Where is it coming from? Is it clear or muffled?

The feeling in the little girl's body, (if you have to go down into the picture and inside the girl's body for a quick association): Where exactly is it? Does it have a size? A temperature? Does it stay the same or does it move at all? Does it have a texture? Is it hard or soft?

Belle is once again dissociated and now changes the picture and the submodalities. For Belle it was all about the finger. She needed some sense of humor there, so in her mind she made the finger very small, much smaller than the rest of the dad's body. She modified the dad's lips and made them smile, she changed his voice to be high-pitched and funny. When she now looked at the picture, still dissociated, it made her smile, she was amused. (I noticed changes in her physiology during the shift of the picture) and when she was once again associated with the little girl, (feeling what she felt, hearing what she heard, seeing what she saw), Belle felt a warm feeling in her body and a sense of peace all over.

Belle no longer "sees" her dad's pointing finger when she eats. In fact, she admits she now feels more comfortable around him, especially when they enjoy family gatherings that involve food.

Barak's encounter with NLP and Physiology of Excellence

We remember 28-year-old Barak, taking his first steps as an acupuncturist and a therapist. Inexperienced and with somewhat low self-esteem and insecure demonstrations of executing his wishes and abilities, Barak embraced the power of NLP as one of the Gymind tools to build up his self-confidence and trust his inner power. Getting him back on track with his physical activity was one way to address the problem. Through running, Barak took control over his body, "got reconnected with his muscles" and felt good about himself. That was one part of the equation, an important one but not sufficient. Our desired outcome was to enable Barak to build up self-confidence, to believe in himself as a gifted acupuncturist and therapist. We wanted him to feel like a successful person, in control of his situation, staying positive and confident no matter what the external circumstances were.

Imagine a ring of power placed on the floor in front of you.

Remember back to a time when you were totally motivated. And when you are feel yourself to be totally motivated, then step into the ring. Barak felt totally motivated when he graduated from school. And also when he won a running competition in the fifth grade. We added additional desired states in the same way: the time when Barak felt totally powerful; when he felt he had tons of energy; when he felt totally loved; when he felt he could have whatever he wanted; a time when he felt totally confident.

When the desired states began to fade, Barak stepped out of the ring.

The same week Barak got three phone calls from potential clients. We have noticed how some things were definitely modified: his walking and posture, the way he sits, the way he speaks - more clearly and more firmly. Without really paying attention, Barak now "owns" a physiology of excellence.

Barak steps into the circle of power each time he needs a boost of energy and confidence.

Anchoring and the power of touch

Research show that physical affection has measurable health benefits. Stimulating touch receptors under the skin can lower blood pressure and cortisol levels, effectively reducing stress (Hertenstein, 2006). A study from the University of North Carolina found that women who hugged their spouse or partner frequently (even for just 20 seconds) had lower blood pressure, possibly because a warm embrace increases oxytocin levels in the brain (Light, 2005). The Department of Nursing from the Umeå University in Sweden found how essential touch is in the process of healing (Edvardsson, 2003). A relationship described as calm, friendly, and humane is created between caregiver and patient when touching is involved, a relationship that transcends the moment of touch and influences one's way of caring. This understanding is presented using the theoretical framework of the philosophy of the existentialist Marcel Gabriel, recognizing that human interaction often involved objective characterization of "the other". Marcel still emphasized the possibility of "communion", a state where both individuals can perceive each other's subjectivity (Marcel, 2007). A hug, a pat on the back, and even a friendly handshake are processed by the reward center in the central nervous system, which is why they can have a powerful impact on the human psyche, making us feel happiness and joy. It doesn't matter if you're the 'toucher' or the 'touchee'. The more you connect with others, at even the slightest physical level, the happier you'll be (Spechler, 2013). This is what "being in rapport" a la NLP is all about. Creating a sense of collaboration synchronized relationship, some intimacy with the patient, in order to help him create a change. The therapist, through "matching and mirroring," gently leads the patient to see shifts and transformations.

In NLP our desirable outcome is to anchor a state in a person, at any time in any modality. We anchored Barak, for instance, when he wished to get reconnected with his sense of confidence and abilities. He was "anchored" into his "Ring of Power". We use anchoring any time a person is in an associated intense state. If at the peak of that experience, a specific stimulus is applied, then the two will be linked neurologically. Anchoring can assist in gaining access to past states and linking the past state to the present and the future (Stevenson, 2007).

The process of anchoring includes four steps:

Have the person recall a past vivid experience.

Anchor (or provide) a specific stimulus at the peak.

Change the person's state.

Evoke the state and set off the anchor to test.

Aida's anchor for running

As we recall from Chapter One, when Aida was 19 years old, she was suffering from excruciating pains in her leg. An ultrasound showed a benign tumor in her thigh. After a successful operation and months in a cast, Aida thought pain was behind her. One day, casually leaning on that operated thigh, she suddenly heard a cracking noise coming from her body, and she found herself on the flour with a broken thigh. Then Aida went though some more painful surgical episodes that left her, until today, with a long nail in her thigh and a broken spirit, almost unable to trust her body. When she came to my studio, determined to lose some weight, Aida mentioned her dream was to run again (25 years after that painful episode). It was at that same meeting that we went out for a first short promising run, enabling Aida to start trusting her body yet again after so many years.

In order to make Aida more confident about taking a good run after the traumatic events she had experienced as a young woman, the anchoring technique was a huge help. Not only did it help Aida achieve a rapport with those great carefree times before her painful episode, but it was an important stimulus that linked neurologically the running in the present and the joy she had felt about it in the past. Every time Aida went for a run, especially in the beginning of her Gymind process, she applied our anchoring method and felt reassured and positive. All it took was to bring together her two fingers, the pointing finger and her thumb, and she would be "anchored" to that good experience.

Can you remember a time when you were totally active, running, maybe winning at a running competition? "Yes, I was 16 or 17 years old, having fun with my friends, feeling carefree and empowered."

As you go back to that time now… go back to that time, float down into your body, and see what you saw, hear what you heard, and really feel the feeling of being totally active.

Now attach your pointing finger to your thumb and make that past activity even greater, more empowering. Multiple that feeling by 10, by 100, by 1000, by million… try to breathe the same way you did then. And feel that experience in your fingers, take a deep breath and come back to now.

It's important to be aware of the sense of touch. Just as we are aware of the physical activity we carry out so that muscles operate better, as we learned in Chapter One, or to be aware of the foods we are eating to make them taste better. Awareness, the power of the conscious mind, is the key to connecting to those subconscious areas: sensations, emotions, blood pressure, health. We are constantly "anchored": we touch the pen we love to write with, and we charge and recharge it with that energy of writing, creating, producing and drawing. We are "anchored" to our children, thanks to those endless hugs that make us feel better, loved, wanted. A touch, any touch charged with emotion, makes us anchored to that emotion. So when you touch the dumbbells at the gym and you enjoy the sensation and the hard work, the next time you touch those dumbbells you are likely to feel the same way. Some people can't bear the touch of running shoes on their feet since they constantly recall or feel how much they hated to run during gymnastics class at school. Be aware of the power of "anchoring" and you can recreate, or better yet manipulate, better experiences by touch. For instance, take your running shoes with you and wear them on your next vacation.

Communication through representational system; Virginia Satir and Milton Erikson

"Anchoring" and many of those mind techniques considered fundamental to the NLP founders, Bandler and Grinder, were derived from the initial modeling of the work of Virginia Satir, an American author and psychotherapist, known especially for her approach to family therapy and her work with family reconstruction. Satir's work was considered pioneering in family practice, in the sense of working at the same time with several members of the same family, instead of with each and every one separately. (Banmen, 2002). Satir identified each member's linguistics patterns and submodalities and "translated" them to the other member of the family in order to create balanced communication and better understanding. According to Satir, negative family scripts could be changed by learning to communicate with feelings. It was her vision for people to realize their self-worth, get back in touch with their feelings, and free themselves from blocked emotions. (Ward, 2012).

"I'm fortunate in being one of the people who pushed my way through to know that people are really round. That's what it means to me to look at people as people who have potential that can be realized, as people who can have dreams and have their dreams work out. What people bring to me in the guise of problems are their ways of living that keep them hampered and pathologically oriented. What we're doing now is seeing how education allows us to move toward more joy, more reality, more connectedness, more accomplishment and more opportunities for people to grow" (Satir, 2012).

Satir's greatness lies in the fact that she realized how each member of the family holds his own representational system preference, and yet they all may face misunderstanding and destructive communicating. Satir, a "mediator" between all parts of the family, identified four representational systems, as summed up by Stevenson (2007):

VISUAL: They memorize by seeing pictures and are less distracted by noise. They are interested by how the program looks. They use predicates such as: see; look; view; appear; show; reveal; picture; hazy; crystal; imagine.

AUDITORY: They are easily distracted by noise, they learn by listening, they like music and like to talk on the phone. The tone of voice and the words they use can be important. They use predicates such as: hear; listen; sound(s); harmonize; unhearing; resonate; silence; rings a bell; be all ears.

KINESTHETIC: They often talk slowly and breathily. They respond to physical rewards and touching. They memorize by doing or walking through something. They will be interested in a program that feels right or gives them a gut feeling. They use predicates such as: feel; touch; grasp; catch on; tap into; concrete; solid; scrape; make contact; get a hold on.

AUDIO-DIGITAL: They spend a fair amount of time talking to themselves. They memorize by steps, procedures, sequences. They will want to know that the program makes sense, and they can also exhibit characteristics of other representational systems. They use predicates such as: sense; experience; understand; think; learn; decide; change; know; distinct; perceive; consider; motivate.

According to the Gymind method, knowing yourself in the sense of your representational system is important for your health. When we know what "type" we are, we may conduct better "dialogues" with ourselves; chose the right words to motivate us, to empower us. We can identify our spouse's internal representational system and create a better rapport with them and better communication with what we referred to as the "outer world".

Barak's language vs. his wife's: Translation for better communication

One of Barak's main goals when he decided to adopt the Gymind way was to interact better with his wife. In fact, he needed to decide whether to stay married and work on some problems they were facing or to leave and break up the famiky. (No kids in the picture yet). Barak wished to begin the Gymind process without his wife, at least for the first sessions. So at first I received "his side of the story", and I was exposed to many dark text messages they had been sending one another for weeks. It was crystal clear how Barak was the kinesthetic type. He needed the touch, the warmth, the cuddle. His choice of words showed how unloved he felt and how his intuition guided his way of thinking, often misguiding his choices. His wife, on the other hand, was more of the auditory, maybe even the audio-digital type. Everything she wrote in those text messages made him angry and frustrated. She used "logic" and "sense", talking about how things don't sound "normal" for her. Through the words I heard her cry for appreciation and understanding. All Barak heard was complaints and alienation. They were both misunderstood, they were both miserable.

A whole system of "translation" was needed there. Barak "learned" a different language in order to communicate better with his wife, but he also gained some clarity in his own mind. Things made sense, he was able to smile again and make better personal choices for himself regarding his career and his physical health.

Barak learned to communicate better with his clients and as a result grew up to be a better therapist, for himself and for others.

Take the representational system preference test: Kinesthetic, visual, auditory and audio-digital. What type are you?

People are situated in different categories to communicate. 40% are Visual, another 40% are Kinesthetic and 20% are Auditory or Auditory Digital. People from different categories will choose their words accordingly. A good therapist will choose the right words in a session in order to be a better communicator and gain rapport. Where are you situated?

For each of the following statements, place a number next to every phrase. Use the following system to indicate your preferences. (Stevenson, 2007):

4 = Closest to describe you

3 = Next best description

2 = Next best

1 = Least descriptive of you

I make important decisions based on:

__ gut level feelings (K)

__ which may sound the best (A)

__ what looks best for me (V)

__ precise review and study of the issues (Ad)

During an argument, I am most likely to be influenced by:

__ the other person's tone of voice (A)

__ whether or not I can see the other person's point of view (V)

__ the logic of the other person's argument (Ad)

__ whether or not I am in touch with the other person's true feelings (K)

I most easily communicate what is going on with me by:

__ the way I dress and look (V)

__ the feeling I share (K)

__ the words I choose (Ad)

__ my tone of voice (A)

It is easiest for me to:

__ find the ideal volume and tuning on a stereo system (A)

__ select the most intellectually relevant point in an interesting subject (Ad)

__ select the most comfortable furniture (K)

__ select rich, attractive color combinations (V)

__ I am very attuned to the sounds of my surroundings (A)

__ I am very adept at making sense of new facts and data (Ad)

__ I am very sensitive to the way articles of clothing feel on my body

(K)

__ I have a strong response to colors and the way a room looks (V)

Step 1: Copy your answers from the previous page to here:

__K __ A __ v __ Ad

__ A __v __Ad __K

__V __K __ Ad __ A

__A __Ad __K __v

__A __Ad __K __V

Step 2: Add the numbers associated with each letter. There are 5 entries for each letter.

	V	A	K	Ad
1				
2				
3				
4				
5				
Totals:				

Step 3: The comparison of the total scores in each column will give the relative preference for each of the four major representational systems.

Convey a message: Hypnosis and hypnotherapy

The Gymind method is about better communication for better health. Not only in its common sense from the Latin commūnicāre, "to share", or the activity of conveying information between two or more people, (Harper, 2013), but also a personal communication in the sense of conveying a message to yourself through the exchange of thoughts, messages, as by speech, visuals, signals, writing, or behavior. We first listen to our bod's needs, become attentive to our thoughts, and then we are able to better communicate with others. In the field of Discourse Analysis and Argumentation, Michel Foucault[6], a 20th century French philosopher, believed that mind control is more powerful than physical punishment in establishing social control, for example (Derrida, 1978). The power of the mind for self-control is critical for a better society. Conveying a message to the self in a certain way determines the mental and physical health of the self. Choice of words, choice of thoughts, choice of certain behaviors are all part of a self-communicational system that defines who we are, how we act and how we feel. Can it be controlled? Altered? Cognitively modified?

Hypnosis is one of those methods for self-communication and alternation of states. It's a natural state that each of us has the ability to enter. Our conscious mind is the part of us that we "think" with. It consists of all of our conscious thoughts, while our subconscious handles the many millions of details that we encounter every day of our life. Basically, hypnosis allows us to open the subconscious mind to suggestions while the conscious mind wanders, or is otherwise distracted (Stevenson, 2004).

Hypnotherapy is a cooperative activity, which requires the full consent of the client. However, all hypnosis is self-hypnosis since the subject enters hypnosis of his own accord. We have all been hypnotized: When we read a book and lose track of all time and feel as though we are 'there'; when we drive down the road and suddenly

---

6 Michel Foucault, (1926-1984) historian of ideas, social theorist, philologist and literary critic, whose theories addressed the relationship between power and knowledge, and how they are used as a form of social control through societal institutions. (Foucault, 1972).

"snap to" ,wondering how we travelled the last few kilometers. These are altered-states where our subconscious mind has jumped to the surface and taken over while our conscious mind wanders. We have talked in Chapter One about the inner elevator that goes occasionally up or down from the conscious to the subconscious or from the subconscious to the conscious. That's the kind of communication that hypnotherapy enables us. We can control, modify, and alter what we have referred to as the "Automaton" for better health. Hypnosis is not in itself a cure for anything. It's a tool, and a very powerful one since it allows the practitioner to speak directly to the subconscious mind. This part is called "intervention" and it's what we say in this part that is most important. As opposed to those affirmations we have encountered in Chapter One, talking to the subconscious mind is as effective as it can get to achieve our goal. A study from the University of California in San Francisco found that hypnosis would be more effective in helping smokers quit than standard behavioral counseling (Carmody, 2008). A study from the University of Frankfurt found that prior clinical hypnosis and NLP have similar success rates of External Cephalic Version procedures[7] and are both superior to standard medical care alone (Reinhard, 2012). Meta-analysis was performed on 18 studies in which a cognitive-behavioral therapy was compared with the same therapy supplemented by hypnosis. The results indicated that the addition of hypnosis substantially enhanced treatment outcome, so that the average client receiving cognitive-behavioral hypnotherapy showed greater improvement than at least 70% of clients receiving non-hypnotic treatment. Effects seemed particularly pronounced for treatments of obesity, especially at long-term follow-up, indicating that unlike those in non-hypnotic treatment, clients to whom hypnotic inductions had

---

7 External cephalic version is a procedure used to turn a fetus from a side-lying (transverse) position into a head-down (vertex) position before labor begins. When successful, version makes it possible for you to try a vaginal birth. (WebMD, 2013).

been administered continued to lose weight after treatment ended (Kirsch, 1995). Randomized controlled studies with clinical populations indicate that hypnosis has a reliable and significant impact on acute procedural pain and chronic pain conditions. Methodological issues of this body of research are discussed, as are methods to better integrate hypnosis into comprehensive pain treatment (Patterson, 2005). One significant study examined the effect of adding hypnosis to a behavioral weight-management program on short and long term weight change. 109 subjects, who ranged in age from 17 to 67, completed a behavioral treatment either with or without the addition of hypnosis. At the end of the 9-week program, both interventions resulted in significant weight reduction. However, at the 8-month and 2- year follow-ups, the hypnosis clients showed significant additional weight loss, while those in the behavioral treatment exhibited little further change. More of the subjects who used hypnosis also achieved and maintained their personal weight goals (Bolocofsky, 1985).

Gymind very often meets people who wish to lose weight. The initial reaction might be to suggest to the subconscious mind "from now on you will eat less". This may seem acceptable to me, but I am using my conscious mind. To the subconscious mind "eating less" is not specific enough, it's too vague. The subconscious mind may interpret this as "from now on I will only eat once a week." A better hypnotic message would be: "From now on you will only have the urge for healthy foods; fatty foods like chocolate and candy will only be eaten moderately or on special occasions. You will decide when your meal is done based purely upon need and fullness…" (Stevenson, 2004).

Milton Erickson was a psychologist and a psychiatrist who truly understood how to communicate with the subconscious minds of others. He was known to use metaphors to convey messages, hypnotize, and heal. A metaphor in this setting is a type of story that has specific, personal, and therapeutic meaning in relation to the subject. Metaphors are usually short stories that when interpreted on a subconscious level give new resources or solutions to the subject (Stevenson, 2004). The subconscious mind is naturally very abstract and metaphorical. The therapeutic metaphor is not a story that is meant to be understood by the conscious mind. On the contrary, it is usually designed to confuse and misdirect the conscious mind while the subconscious mind draws parallels and derives meanings from the story in relation to its current dilemmas.

When Barak questioned his relationship with his wife, he felt at times trapped in a somewhat abusive relationship. In a process of "metaphor and storytelling" I casually "confused" his conscious mind with a story about my late grandma who escaped from a prison camp in World War II. It was a short story, yet it gave Barak's subconscious mind the perspective it needed to evoke a healthy attitude so he could focus on the good memories he had been sharing with his wife. Needless to say, he is still married and enjoys a good relationship with his beloved wife.

Oliver, the formerly hypotonic child whom we met in previous chapter, heard the story about Milton Erickson who was paralyzed but with the help of great will power and lots of training, swimming, mind games and self-belief, learned to walk again (Haley, 1993). For the former hypotonic kid, this was a great inspiration to overcome his own physical difficulties. Oliver also loves to hear stories about other kids who encounter Gymind. Hearing about other boys and girls his age encourages him to keep on going, inspires him to eat right, and keep on with his strength training. Oliver often compares his progress to the progress of other kids he does not know in person, obviously, but can relate to their stories, their disabilities, and their motivation to achieve better health.

Being at Hakalau and using "the third eye"

Hakalau, or Peripheral vision, is a physical and mental state of BEING, present in the present. Being at Hakalau means "to stare at as in meditation and to allow to spread out" (ancientHuna.com). It's a very ancient technique derived from martial arts from Hawaii, when fighters were trained how to use their mind for full awareness in order to fight four, five or six people at the same time and even to know when someone was behind them. Hakalau is the means in the ancient Hawaiian system for entering a rapid trance state at will.

We normally use our five senses. This particular sense belongs to the area of the "third eye", the intuitive vision, that resides in the middle of our forehead. Hakalau can be a real eye-opener, taking everything that's distracting out of the system. There are millions of bits of information entering our system at any given moment. But in fact because of our filter system we can name only a few. When we are in the peripheral vision, we are aware of everything. We can see what's actually happening at any given time. (NLPWorld.co.uk). We expand our abilities to see, we pass over boundaries as the conscious mind grasps them. Milton Erickson likes to describe therapy as a way of helping people to extend their limits (Haley, 1993).

Pick a spot on the wall to look at, preferably above eye level, so that your field of vision seems to bump up against your eyebrows, but the eyes are not so high so as to cut off the field of vision.

Let go. As you stare at this spot, just let your mind go loose, and focus all of your attention on the spot.

Spread out. Notice that within a matter of moments your vision begins to spread out, and you see more in the peripheral than you do in the central part of your vision.

Pay attention to the peripheral. In fact, pay more attention to the peripheral than to the central part of your vision.

Stay in this state for as long as you can. Notice how it feels. Notice the ecstatic feelings that begin to come to you as you continue the state.

Expend your awareness further and further. Go across the wall of the room. Go all the way and try to hear the sound of the sea, people on the shore; the sound of cars outside. See how far you can go with that awareness. And then there is nothing else but your awareness. You are present, you are here but you are not in your filter system. That's when you know someone is thinking about you or when you are thinking about someone and he calls you. You can talk in hakalau. You don't have to know what you say and it just goes out there intuitively and releases you. Hakalau allows you to know beyond your normal knowledge.

Ave's applications of hakalau

Ave, 31, married with a 1-year-old child, has been a dear client of mine for over four years now, since way back before she was married. We are currently working on shedding baby fat and bringing her back to her balanced weight of 64 kg. One of her many obstacles is eating at night, especially when she brings work home with her, since she is obliged to accomplish long late hours in front of her computer. That's when she needs to take a bite, supposedly in order to make her more alert, concentrated, and productive. However, because of those late night snacks, her weight would not budge. During our weekly running sessions, I asked Ave some questions, to which all the answers were "Yes": 1. Do you work in the kitchen? 2. Are you facing the kitchen cabinets and/or the refrigerator? 3. Do you work late after having eaten a good dinner? We concluded that: 1. Ave was "anchored" to the sensation of eating while she was working. She sat on that chair in the kitchen, in front of that table in the kitchen, an environment that did not match the energy of working. 2. Logistically Ave could not work elsewhere. But while Ave thinks that's all she sees, (the computer, the screen, the words she writes, her hands and maybe the table), her senses are at Hakalau, and so she constantly absorbs all there is in the kitchen. We then decided she would turn her back to the kitchen while working. Turning her back to the kitchen cabinets, and when her mind is now at Hakalau, Ave perceives other signals: the living room, the windows, other objects in the room, but not food and everything related to it. The next morning I got this short text message saying: "Sometimes you really succeed in amazing me. I worked three hours last night with my back to the kitchen cabinets, drinking nothing but warm tea and needed no food at all!".

Rapport, better communication and Self Alternation during physical training

A good communicator must build a rapport with his client. Rapport is all about working together; it's a "do with" process with the client as opposed to "do to" process. It's meant to be subtle and at the subconscious level. In NLP, rapport is a process as opposed to hypnosis, where it's a state. (Stevenson, 2008).

Back in 2007, in LA, I approached my trainer and teacher at the time, Michael Stevenson, and asked him with some concern: "I often work with clients, not necessarily while we sit on comfortable chairs like when we practice here, but I train them physically. I jog when they need to jog, I lift weights when they need to, I am constantly exercising with them during our session. Can I create a rapport? Can I help them achieve their mental health using NLP techniques and everything we learn here?" Stevenson gave me a profound, somewhat sympathetic look and answered without hesitation: "You might do even better, much better for communicating with your clients and with constructing a rapport when you do everything with them". He then gathered the class and listed five things to match in getting rapport. Physiology: matching our breathings, steps; Tonality, tempo, timbre or range of voice; Choice of Words: Match predicates to get rapport; matching key words, common experience and associations. When we move the same way as our client does, we are into the "cross-over mirroring" technique, as we match at least one part of the subject's physiology with another part of ours. We get into a "pace, pace, lead; pace, pace, lead" rhythm; we hence gain rapport and full attention from the subject.

We also aim to keep it possible to talk and to convey ideas during physical sessions, according to the "rate of perceived exertion" scale created by Gunnar Borg, referred to as the "Borg Scale". It offers major benefits:

Connecting mind and body.

Assessing the perception of how hard you are working.

Allowing the trainer to more clearly communicate how difficult a specific exercise should "feel" (Borg, 1982).

A study from the Department of Exercise and Sport Science UW- La Crosse confirms the robust relationship between ventilatory threshold and the "Talk Test" during various interventions, suggesting that the talk test is suitable for prescribing exercise (Foster, 2008).

Rate of perceived exertion based on the talk test:

1-2 (light): You can talk easily

3 (Moderate): You can chat comfortably.

> When the client is at 1-3 level we exchange ideas, bring up the problem, learn about the client's personal history and understand what we are about to be working on mentally.

4-5 (Moderately tough): Chatting is taking much more effort.

6-7 (Tough): More difficult to sustain a conversation.

8-9 (Very difficult): It takes a lot of effort to chat.

> When the client is at 4-9 level, it's up to me to begin and create change through metaphors, representational systems, imagination, and the power of words. At that level the conscious mind is distracted, so that the conversation I manage is

mostly with the subconscious mind. Shifts are made, learnings are created.

10 (Maximum effort): No talking, only focus.

A Gymind session and verbal and behavioral communication while training outdoors can be a spiritual experience. Five years ago I began to work with 40-year-old Jonathan, who confided to me he was still a virgin looking for a female partner, someone to hold and love. Jonathan also needed to lose some weight and to eat smart. We had experienced some exciting Gymind sessions together. Not only did Jonathan lose 10 kilograms of his body fat and adopted better nutritional habits, but he also made significant mental progress regaining confidence and a better body image. We practiced his social communication skills till Jonathan was ready to approach a woman and introduce himself. I remember one significant session when we went outside for a 5-km. run. It was a cool, calm night. At 10 p.m. it was only Jonathan and I jogging along an empty road. It was then and there that we practiced the Hakalau technique. While running we got a peripheral vision of that beautiful road that seemed to progress in an opposite direction to ours, making it seem as if we were running faster than we actually were. It was a thrilling metaphor of our life, how days go by faster than anyone can grasp. It started to rain, gently. This was a perfect moment to create this beautiful thought about how the rain was washing off all the doubts, fears, and uncertainties in Jonathan's life. As I sensed Jonathan's physical effort and his rapid breathing, I knew his subconscious mind got reconnected to the scenery, bonding with nature, planting at that moment the seeds of competence, capabilities, and inner strength that Jonathan needed so badly.

Two years later Jonathan found his soul mate and got married.

Time Line Therapy: Finding your time line for a deep change

"The Secret" (Byrne, 2006) is one of those inspirational books and movies. It talks about the "law of attraction" and how we can summon abundance, create a better life for ourselves and maintain impeccable health using the power of our mind. The primary thought of "taking faith in our own hands using our mind" is groundbreaking yet prominent and influential, so that millions of people rushed to buy the book and discover the secret. Oprah gave it a platform on her talk-show and it was the "book of the hour" for a long time, maybe even until today. The only problem with "The Secret" is that it left out a lot of substance. For Gymind, it's only an introduction and not a complete lesson on the art and skill of manifestation. Where "Doing" is not complete without the "Being"; where Body goes hand in hand with Mind; when fitness and nutrition are not enough to maintain one's health. With "The Secret" people mistakenly thought all they had to do was "ask, believe, and receive," and life would magically change instantly. It didn't. And just as we cannot put a 100 piece puzzle together if we have 10 pieces missing, something was missing in this great and powerful theory.

It was 'Time Line Therapy', the model, the practice, the technique in order to achieve transformation and even change of personality. Our Time Line is the memory coding of the brain. It is how people encode and store their memories. With the discovery of Time Line we have, for the first time, the ability to change a significant number of a person's memories in a short time. Obviously changing a substantial number of a person's memories will have an impact on the person's personality (Tad James, 1988).

Time Line Therapy techniques began as a part of the field of NLP and contain elements of NLP and hypnotic language. As a model it has the potential to not only make sense out of our temporal experience, but also to change our understanding of how negative emotions and limiting decisions affect us, as well as describing how to create a meaningful future for all time to come, because with Time Line Therapy we now understand the human temporal experience and can change the basic elements that make up someone's history.(Stevenson, 2007).

The Time Line Therapy techniques may be a relatively recent development. However, the idea of an individual having the means of knowing the difference between memories of the past and the future, or having a "Time Line" is not. William James wrote in 1890 his theory that the subconscious mind stores memories in linear time in his "principles of Psychology". He based this theory on Aristotle who was one of the first in our culture to mention the idea of a "Time Line" in Physics IV, (1957), for the Greeks had a clear idea of temporality. "Western minds represent time as a straight line upon which we stand with our gaze directed forward; before us we have the future and behind us the past. On this line we can unequivocally define all tenses by means of points. The present is the point on which we are standing, the future is found on some point in front of us and in between lies the exact future; behind us lies the perfect, still farther back the imperfect and farther yet the pluperfect." According to Aristotle we must represent time by the image of a line or by the image of movement along a line, either a circular line or a straight line.

This is where we take the journey to the collection of our memories, recorded and stored, as we age and with time they have more and more influence (Tad James, 1988). Time as a mental construct and neuro-linguistic representation can allow us to transfer experience and represent time the way we choose.

Anglo-European time describes "time" in terms of one event happening after another. It sees time as linear and the events stretching out like an assembly line. A person characterized by the Anglo-European concept of time will seek to arrive "on time".

Arabic time describes an entirely different approach. A person acting by the Arabic concept of time will rarely arrive in such a timely manner. People from the Islamic countries and areas of the world with warm climates live primarily in Arabic time. They live the moment.

In fact, a time line may move out in any direction and may take all kinds of forms and shapes: as a straight line, a spiral, a loop, a boomerang. One of my client's time line begins in front of her as a straight line and then goes all the way up into the endless skies. The line may direct your body "in time" or move around and outside your body "through time". "Through-time" people usually dissociate from their memories and so see themselves in their memories. An "in-time" person will more likely have their time "past" behind them. Because "in-time" people associate inside of "time", they can get "lost in the eternal now" and have no idea "what time it is" (Bodenhamer, 1998).

We meet people about whom we think "she is living in the past" or "all he thinks about is the future; he never takes time to stop and smell the roses" or "she only lives for today; she has no conception of where she is going". These qualities are determined by the ways people represent time internally. The ways people represent time: past, future, present, provide the basis for their skills and limitations. Because of this, it is impossible to fix some problems unless you change a person's way of representing time (Andreas, 1987).

When Jonathan came to my studio 5 years ago, he was having phobias and fears, low self-esteem, lack of confidence and minimum sense of control over the course of his life. We immediately identified his "time-line". His past was directed ahead of him and his future – behind him. Subconsciously his past was always ahead, blocking his future, so that Jonathan was constantly living in the past. "Jonathan", I asked, intrigued. "Does it make sense to you that your past is in front of you?" "Yes, it does. It feels normal to me". "Can we change your time line and place the future in front of you? If it's not comfortable we will change it back to the way it was. Is that ok with you?" "Yes, it is", Jonathan said.

It was only after we moved the past-line behind him in order to "put things in the past" and moved the future-line in front of him "to enable him to lead his life experiences to the future that awaits for him, that Jonathan could continue freely with his life, no longer "haunted" by his past.

"It's never too late to have a happy childhood" (Richard Bandler)

Richard Bandler's statement, "It is never too late to have a happy childhood" (Bandler, 1985), is the key to de-energize old hurtful memories and to access numerous resources for venturing more joyfully and lovingly through "time" (Bodenhamer, 1998). "Time" does not exist in that dimension of reality. It rather exists in the realm of "mind". It refers to a conceptual way of marking a process as events transpire and between events that occur. The proper place of words in our life is to help us keep track of our experiences, by labeling them and categorizing them (Andreas, 1987). We can then "call up" an experience when it's useful to us, modify it, shift it, learn, and accept new skills and new information. The words on a menu bring up the taste and texture of the food described. The words are not the food, they point to the food. We use words to create new taste, new memories.

Discover your time line and take your first adventure

I have a feeling that if I were to ask your subconscious mind, "where is your future and where is your past?" that you'd point in a certain direction, like front to back, side to side, up and down, or in some direction in relation to your body. Now it's not your conscious, logical, thought-out answer that I want, it's your natural, unconscious answer I want, your first impulse. So if I were to ask your unconscious mind, where is your future? what direction would you point? Good. And where is your past? Notice those directions imply a line"

What I'd like you to do now is this: just go ahead and close your eyes, and think of your timeline. Now when I say timeline, I don't really mean something you see, because in a moment I am going to ask you to float above it, and by float, I also mean as sound waves float on the wind, or as you might float in a pool or bathtub. So go ahead now and just float above your timeline, making sure to look through your own eyes, instead of seeing your own self floating. I'd like you now to just turn and face the past and just float right back into the past as far as you'd like and give me a nod when you are there. Good. Now go ahead and turn around back towards now, facing the future, and just go ahead and float right out into the future and give me a nod when you are there. Good. Now turn around and face now, so you're facing back into the past. And now I want you to float way up into the air. In fact, float so high that your entire timeline seems to be only a centimeter long. And when you are there, just go ahead and float all the way back down to now and come back into the room (Stevenson, 2007).

Discovering and connecting to our personal timeline is the basis and core of therapy. It gives perspective, a new point of view, combined with the ability to summon up memories, events, traumas from the past and deal with them while dissociated and to recreate them, differently; without the sting, without the shock and without the pain.

So the next step would be to find the root cause, the first significant event that needs to be modified. Discovering the line is only the beginning.

Transparency in therapy

My personal discovery of the root cause was a defining moment as a person and as a therapist. A true "WOW moment" as Oprah often puts it. This was a real eye-opener as far as how much Mind and Body are connected, and it really gave a pure personal therapy as a bonus. We are about to dive into that significant moment; however, it aroused a major question concerning transparency in counseling and in therapy: Should Gymind personal experiences be revealed during sessions? Certainly, it will help with creating a rapport with the client, a mutual understanding, and empathy on both sides. But is it the right way? Shouldn't Gymind simply and totally lead the client to find his own path and to create his own story line without a potential overload of personal experiences and private revelations?

Discussions of psychotherapist self-disclosure date back to the earliest years of psychotherapy. As early as 1912 Freud emphasized that "The physician should be impenetrable to the patient and like a mirror, reflect nothing but what is shown to him" (Petersen, 2002). The rise of the humanist movement in the 60s advanced the argument that self-disclosure could be therapeutic and valuable. In 1971 Jourard published "Self-disclosure: An Experimental Analysis of the Transparent Self", which has been highly popular among humanistic psychotherapists ever since. The feminist movement of the 1970s and 1980s added a political dimension, in which feminist therapist self-disclosure was valued for its role in modeling a more egalitarian relationship between therapist and client (Simi, 1997). Simultaneously, the 12-step programs used in many support groups, which are based on mutual self-disclosure, have proliferated since the 1980s and 1990s. The 1990s have witnessed a cultural shift where celebrities and politicians, such as Oprah Winfrey, Kitty Dukakis, Elizabeth Taylor, and Patty and Michael Reagan, have accustomed the public to intimate and detailed confessions on national TV. In the new millennium, so-called reality shows that promote uncensored voyeurism and uninhibited self-disclosure have burgeoned (Zur, 2011). I found over the years that stories and metaphors a la Milton Erickson are so influential that I was willing, compelled, and obliged to reveal and share pertinent parts of my own story for a wholesome and sincere purpose, when the time was right to do so. Clients hear stories about other clients (they don't know) and become inspired. We perceive this current book as a revelation of case-studies and personal encounters with the self and create a whole thesis out of it, of how to Gymind your way in life.

Discover the root cause, a personal WOW moment to share

It was way back in 2007. I was in Los Angeles, California, learning about the secrets and wonders of NLP and Time Line, when I began to practice with a partner how to discover the root cause of anger. My partner Tim, whom I had never met before this class, was sitting in front of me with the Time Line script on his lap. He did not seem too confident, being a student himself playing the role of a therapist, but I knew I had to trust whatever answer came out of my mouth since it was the subconscious mind's doing and not my thinking. I trusted the words, the answers that came out without giving them much thought.

Is it all right with your unconscious mind for you to release this anger and for you to be consciously aware of it now?

"Yes" I answered.

Good. Ask your unconscious, what is the root cause of this problem which, when disconnected, will cause the problem to totally disappear? If you were to know, was it before, during or after your birth?

"Before" my subconscious quickly answered.

Good. Was it in the womb, or before that?

"In the womb," I said.

Good, what month in the womb?

"Seventh".

Tim continued:

Just go ahead and get in touch with your time line now. Float above your timeline and turn around and face the past. And go ahead and float back into the past to the point where you can see the event from the side, right before it happened, to position number 1. And when you get there, just notice the event and give me a nod.

I nodded. I did not see anything but I felt I was there. (I have already identified myself as being kinesthetic).

Now float to position number 2, directly over the event and looking down on it. Ask your unconscious mind what it needs to learn from this event, the learning of which will allow you to let go of the anger, easily and effortlessly. Your unconscious mind can preserve these learnings so that if it needs them in the future, they will go there to protect you. You may get learnings consciously or you may just get an indication that you've gotten them. When you've got the learning, please let me know".

I then heard myself saying: "I am strong; I can do whatever I want".

At that moment I was still "playing the game". I still did not see anything, I simply followed Tim's instructions. At that point I could only hope that I did everything right.

Now go ahead and float to position number 3, turning around to see the future, so that the event is in front of you and below you. And ask yourself: Now, where is the anger? Is it there or is it gone now?

Now float right down to the event so you are looking through your own eyes. Now check on the anger. Is it there or is it gone? Good. Go back to position number 3.

Now come back to now over your timeline only as quickly as you can let go of all the anger all the way back to now. Stop at position number 3, preserve the learnings, and let go of all the anger all the way back to now. And when you get back to now, go ahead and float down into now and come back into the room.

As I was floating back on my timeline, I felt a brief caressing touch on my left clavicle all the way to my left shoulder. I quickly opened my eyes to see whether Tim or anybody else was touching me, but it was nothing really; only this wonderful physical sensation of a magical caress, a "load off" of my chest, a sense of liberation. I raised my arm and called Michael to join Tim and me in order to explain what I had just felt. Stevenson confirmed that the physical impact after having discovered the root cause and having accepted those learnings is varied from one person to another, but that a physical impact is definitely there.

That physical relief I experienced consisted of mental events that were unconsciously there for so many years: At 7 months in the womb I encountered my mom's anger, fears, and pain since she had to stay in bed throughout her pregnancies to keep her embryos alive. My parents had lost their firstborn child, delivered ahead of time at week 27th and died at the age of 10 days. My parents were experiencing a mixture of negative emotions that I absorbed as a fetus. As a 34-year-old woman, my conscious mind had nothing to do with all that. But my subconscious mind definitely did.

The physical caress I experienced was only the beginning. Several months later I rechecked my blood pressure, a regular routine for me, since I have been genetically suffering since forever from high blood pressure; nothing that required medical involvement, but definitely surveillance and monthly follow-ups. To my amazement, measurements were normal and have stayed normal ever since.

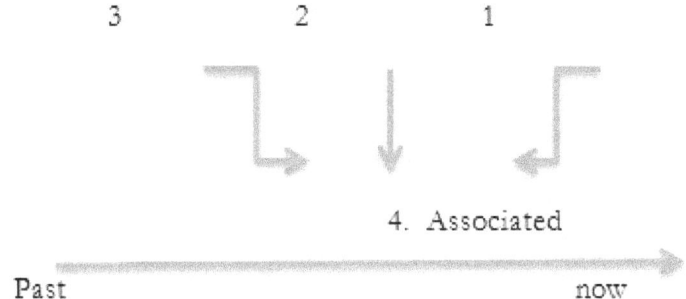

Maya's time line

We remember Maya's heart condition at birth, so that when she consulted her cardiologist about her wish to become a mom, he ordered her to get in shape and to lose some weight. That was the reason for our longstanding productive encounters. Time went by, Maya achieved her physical goals, and after several trials to get pregnant and two rounds of IVF treatments, she gave birth to two healthy babies, a boy and a girl, Guy and Roni, on March 20th 2013. During delivery, things did not go smoothly. Maya's heart almost did not make it, and she almost died of heart failure. When Maya was 6 months pregnant, she and her husband moved to the north of Israel to be closer to her parents. Maya and I lost touch. It was two weeks after the painful and frightening delivery that her husband gave me a call, asking me to start therapy over the phone in order to ease the pain and help Maya's heart to heal.

Timeline therapy is so powerful in the sense of the mind-body connection and the physical permanent shift that it can be experienced over the phone at any time of the day. In Maya's case we were compelled to first rely on the wise philosophy of Yehuda Halevi foremost poet and thinker of the Jewish Middle Ages in his work "The Kuzari". (1139 CE). In the easy format of a Platonic dialogue, it presents a meeting between the ruler of the Khazar kingdom and a Jewish sage, who discuss a series of theological, philosophical and ideological dilemmas that are timely, timeless, and universal. It is there where we find for the first time that the heart is the true home of the soul. It's interesting how anatomically the heart itself cannot get sick. No cancer, viruses, or germs reach the heart. Yet it feels the soul's pain and hence becomes sick: worries, grief, resentments, hatred, fears, they all impact the heart's condition and its health. Even bad nutrition and insufficient hydration can have a bad influence on the heart, says Halevi almost 3000 years ago.

Towards the end of the 19th century, Dr. Butto Nader, a chirurgical cardiologist, emphasizes the importance of the spiritual aspect and seeks knowledge that aims to fill the gaps in conventional medicine. With the Seventh Sense (2004), he developed an energetic method that tracked down emotional conflict (and its state), which caused the energetic block and that eventually evolved as a physical illness. This unique method opens the energetic block and washes the body with a flow of life, energy, and vitality. In matters of the heart, the ancient yet universal philosophy of Halevi and the physical and spiritual methodology of Dr. Butto form a solid belief system that a mental and spiritual approach would help Maya's condition and improve her heart functions.

Maya's timeline therapy became essential and mostly effective after the delivery of her twins and her near-death experience. Her life became so complicated in the months that followed the event: Being a new mom of twins; not being able to take care of them for many weeks; tension in her family and the awakening of old demons from back when she was a baby herself, going under the knife. Combining mental and spiritual therapy with fitness and healthy nutrition was a must, and so the timeline served as a reliable tool for health. Maya has traveled more than a dozen times above and over her timeline. She discovered her Past was in the back; the Future went all the way up to the unlimited skies, bringing, as she pointed, "a sense of growth and hope".

We present here three episodes, three "limiting beliefs" on Maya's timeline.

June 17th, 2010. Two years before the delivery. Finding the root cause of Maya's heart surgery as a baby.

The limiting belief: problems with the left side of the body.

"When did you decide you were having problems in your left side of your body? Was it before, during or after your birth?"

Maya: "In the womb, one week old".

"Go ahead and get in touch with your timeline now. Float above your timeline and turn around and face the past. And go ahead and float back into the past right down into position number four. Right into the event. Notice the limiting decision that occurred there, and notice the emotions too. Give me a nod when you've done that".

Maya did more than that, she told what she saw, felt and heard:

"I see my mother's pregnancy. I am one week old, in the womb. I feel uncomfortable. I recognize worries and doubts".

"Now go ahead and float back into position number 3, turn around and face the future, so you are before the beginning of the event and any of the chains of events that led up to it. Ask your unconscious mind what it needs to learn from this, which will allow it to let go of all the limiting decision, and to let go of the emotions easily and effortlessly. Ask yourself: now where is the decision? Is it there or is it just gone now? And the emotions too".

Maya: "My mom feels uncomfortable, she worries a lot, my dad is in the army, and she is alone. She needs some peace of mind; she needs confidence and mental health to keep her calm".

"Now float right down into the event, so you are looking through your own eyes. Now check on the emotions and the decision. Are they there, or are they just gone now?"

Maya: "They are gone. I know and feel that the problem is no longer mine. It belongs to my mother. I feel peaceful; my body can continue to grow peacefully"

"Good. Go back to position number 3. Now come back to now over your timeline as quickly as you can. Stop at three events along your timeline where, had you never made that limiting decision, you would have had many more opportunities. Stop and notice these three events and watch as they reevaluate themselves in light of these new choices and opportunities. Stop at each event in position number 3, preserve the learnings and let go of the emotions, all the way back to now. Remember, at the unconscious level, there is no concept of time so your unconscious can take as much time or as little time as it wants to. Just let go of the emotions and that limiting belief all the way back to now, and when you get to now, go ahead and float down into now and come back into the room".

Maya did not share her experiences while she was floating beck into the now. It was only after she opened her eyes that she revealed this sensation of pure relief she felt all over her body. She did come across an event that had occurred back when she was 15 years old. She used to have black circles under her eyes, and teenage friends used to ask her about it. She did feel more confident, she did not care when they did this now, on that journey back over her timeline, and things looked much less intimidating and harsh.

May 25th, 2012. Two month after the delivery. Maya first talks about her fears of her near-death experience. She encounters everything from a "floating point of view" which gives her clarity and perspective, but most of all, a chance to embrace her learnings and move on with her life, stronger.

The timeline script remains almost the same; Maya reconnected with her timeline and begins her journey. As Maya floats over her timeline, she tells her story in a calm, deep, relaxed, "hypnotized" voice.

"I am in the hospital, two weeks after delivery. I see the nurse; she allows me to see the babies only from a distance. I feel helpless, sick-to-death. This is the first time I am willing to see the babies. I was reluctant to see pictures or to hear stories about them. My sister-in-law, a child psychologist, called me the day before, suggesting they bring the babies home so that they would not suffer from the lack of a mother figure. Home, this is not an option for me now. My parents have doubts about my abilities to emotionally function as a mom, yet the doctors give me all the time I need to heal and stand on my own two feet. I cannot deal with the idea that I would see them, reconnect with them and then eventually would not be there for them. I have created a wall because I was scared to death, I was afraid I would die. Every time I went to see the babies, I was experiencing palpitations. I was afraid of what my brothers and sister would say or ask. So I rarely went there".

"What are your learnings? Ask your subconscious what does it learn from that?"

Maya continued: "I now remember the day my friend, who had lost her father after a long battle with cancer, came to visit. We could hardly talk because they took me to see the babies, but I now hear her voice loud and clear. She was telling me what a strong wonderful mom I was, how ready I was for motherhood, and how long I had been waiting for this. Her words "we should release our grasp, we cannot control everything" made me stronger. I can focus on Guy and Roni and ignore my brothers and sister who doubted my maternal abilities. I sent an email to my brothers telling them to help me in the way I needed help. I pleaded with them not to ask me whether I had seen the babies or not and why. I reassured them that I was a wonderful mom and that I knew without a shadow of a doubt that I would reconnect with my babies and that I would love them and be there for them forever".

"What are your learnings? Ask your subconscious: what does it learn from that?" I asked again.

Maya received a message from her subconscious mind: "Nonchalance, indifference, strength, love, growth, motherhood, peace and quiet".

She then floated back over her timeline, knowing the palpitations would be experienced less and less, understanding what a powerful mom she is and will be. Maya admitted she was no longer afraid of death; she knows now she is here to stay, stronger than ever, focusing on what matters most. This was a mini-breakthrough that enabled Maya to move on and enjoy her motherhood.

January 14th 2012. Ten months after delivery. Things at home are much better, Maya functions as a mother, her parents help a lot with the babies. Maya feels better, less weak, and her heart's condition improves tremendously.

Maya still experiences palpitations, sometimes four-five times a day. She knows physically how to make it stop, holding her breath for a few moments and looking at her beautiful twins.

The limiting belief: Experiencing palpitations.

"When was it you decided on having palpitations? Was it before, during or after your birth?"

Maya: "Before my birth, in a past life, two lifetimes ago".

"I am in NY City, I see many buildings, it's sunny yet very cold outside. There is a baby in the street, and I don't see his mother anywhere. I feel uncertainty and fear. My heart beats strongly now. The baby does not cry but he looks around, trying to understand why his mother is not coming back. He sees her escaping, running away, she cannot take care of him. She feels awful because she cannot take care of him, and she has no other choice but to run away in the hopes that someone else will take care of him".

"What are your learnings? Ask your subconscious what does it learn from that?"

Maya: "Faith, power, will, daring, courage, choice, power, security, love."

"The picture is changing now. The mother stops and sits down. She is confused. She misses her baby. Her heart is at peace now. Her whole body feels that peace; she walks slowly, contemplating what just happened. She regains more power, more confidence".

Maya chose to paint the woman's throat in blue, representing for her safety and security. She painted her feet and pelvis in red, for energy and sense of control.

I then guide Maya to enter the baby's body. She notices that he is suspicious at first, a bit disappointed and then feels secure and regains his inner strength. When Maya looks from above, she sees harmony and joy. She continues: "Before this lady became pregnant, she was a secretary. She wanted to go back to work, she needed a supporting husband, she needed to be loved. She now gets up, takes the baby in her arms, and goes to search for a job. She becomes a secretary in a high-tech firm and puts her baby in the firm's day care service. She is the receptionist, gets a promotion, she is happy. The baby is close to her".

Floating back over her timeline back to the Maya of now, she knows all of a sudden that she needs to move back to the center of Israel and leave her parents' surroundings, in order to have more peace and quiet and to reduce her palpitations to a minimum.

Aida's time line

When Aida decided more than two years ago to become a runner despite her sad experiences as a 19-year-old woman, nothing was standing in her way, as we learned in Chapter One. Her mental willpower was so strong that her body followed almost instantly and helped her become the runner she had always wished to be. However, when Aida confided in me about her fear of flying and how this fear disabled her for so many years from joining her family on those annual family vacations, or when she did finally get on the plane, it was not without narcotic assistance, we decided to release that fear. One of the tools we decided to work with was, of course,

Time Line Therapy.

We had an obvious root cause for that fear. The traumatic event at the age of 19 took its mental toll on Aida, and we could not avoid the fact that she had never really received any mental support during or after her surgeries, nor years after, up until our Gymind process. Aida's loving parents wished to deliver a strong message that "everything is OK", a wonderful attitude that has helped Aida a lot up until today and strengthened her spirit back then. And yet, the events were apparently too traumatic to treat with positive affirmations or repressions.

Aida's timeline passes through her body. Her past goes down into her feet, and her future continues on a straight line up.

"Just go ahead and get in touch with your time line now. Float above your timeline and turn around and face the past. And go ahead and float back into the past to the point where you can see the event from the side, the traumatic fall you experienced, right before it happened, to position number 1. And when you get there, just notice the event and give me a nod".

Aida: "I see myself after the first surgery, standing in my room next to my closet, trying to pick up an outfit to wear. It's only minutes before the fall, before I break my thigh and before those two other excruciating surgeries".

"Go down into the event and stand in front of that 19-year-old girl. Look at her, wait for her to look at you. This 45-year- old strong and capable runner is standing face to face with the 19-year-old version of her. You want to help. What do you say to her?"

Aida is having some difficulties speaking. She is too choked with emotion. "I am holding her" she says. "I tell her it's ok to be afraid. It's ok to fall down. That she can do it. I give her strength. I give her love and energy. I give her everything I feel when I am running, and everything I experience after a good run. She is listening and smiling. She does not really understand but she listens and smiles. I give her confidence, strength, power, stamina, endurance".

We could not change the course of events. Aida did fall down and broke her thigh. But when the 45-year-old looked at the event now over her timeline it was not traumatic at all. It was an event, empty of fear, vacant of terrible emotions. The situation might be terrifying, but Aida did not sense that any longer. She floated all the way back "free as a bird" as she confessed. The next flight she took several weeks later made her as proud as the first time she accomplished a 2 km run without a single stop.

Changing Aida's timeline

As mentioned earlier, Aida's timeline passes through her body. Her past goes down into her feet, and her future continues a straight line up. Aida agreed to change her timeline and make the past stay in the past, bringing her future to appear in front of her.

"Go ahead and float over your timeline now. Reconnect to your timeline as you perceive it as the long hand of a clock. Extend your arms, reach out and grab that hand and gently move it horizontally, adjusting your timeline to its new orientation, making sure you identify the line of the past and the line of the future. Reconnect to now and float back into the room. Try to feel the past and all your lifetime experiences behind you. Look in front of you and see the line of your future. Make sure it feels right for you".

Irene's timeline

We have met courageous Irene and her fight against Lupus, the fact that she refuses to take any medications yet through fitness and smart nutrition has reduced pain and discomfort resulting from her condition by 90 percent, as she admits. Her mental and spiritual growth is admirable. Right before our eyes, from one training session to the other, Irene has evolved and blossomed. Irene has taken control over her body, the words she was using, her nutrition, her life and has become a changed woman. Time Line Therapy also played a significant role in her recovery. It gave her a new perspective, it taught her subconscious new learnings to the extent that Irene once wrote to me: "I look at people in the street. Walking by, in a hurry, rushing from one place to another, not realizing how deep everything really is, how powerful their mind is and what little use they make of it. This brain of mine is such a powerful tool that I wish to use it more and more". On January 17th, 2011 two weeks into our Gymind process, Irene floated over her timeline back to the traumatic event that triggered Lupus, the birth of her third child. She observed from above and saw that helpless, hopeless, sick women, just lying there hating the world. Irene received several understandings and learnings. Her subconscious provided her with love, happiness, power, life, and the colors white and blue she chose to fill her heart and her throat with. It was on that session that Irene realized she behaved just like her mother had: Always the victim. She realized how much her body misses a tender motherly touch and had been missing that all those years growing up as a kid; that she subconsciously may constantly blame her mother for the lack of it which causes so much tension between them.; tension that does not help her with the process of healing.

Irene and I talked about a television interview with one of the Israel's top comedians, Adir Miller. He was interviewed by the famous psychiatrist, Yoram Yovel, who asked him about the relationship with his parents. This story served as a wonderful metaphor a la Milton Erikson in order to help Irene's health. Miller compared his parent's love to a test in History at school. "When you answer correctly yet write down more than you were asked for, your history teacher marks "X" on those redundant parts but won't reduce your grade. Whereas when your answer is lacking or incomplete you get a low grade for that. My parents gave me too much love and attention, some of it exceeded the level of needs, so I knew to mark "X", yet always felt complete and loved. I know how some kids don't receive that, just like a failing grade in a history test, and they spend their whole life searching for recognition and love out there".

This is how Irene felt about her parents, especially her mother.

Irene has experienced many timeline sessions over the years we have been working together. She floated over her timeline back to a past life, realizing how strong and meaningful the relationship with her husband really is. She has found tenderness in her life, learned to embrace a relationship with other women whose role as "replacement mom" was now accepted and understood. Irene received the key to happiness and has been opening doors with it ever since. Mentally and emotionally, Irene is on the right path.

Governing emotions for a change

We discussed earlier on about the golden age of brain research we are witnessing nowadays. How considerable progress has been made over the past 20 years in relating specific circuits of the brain to emotional functions. Much of this work has involved studies of Pavlovian or classical fear conditioning, a behavioral procedure that is used to couple meaningless environmental stimuli to emotional (defense) response networks. This is very much like the "anchoring" technique we have encountered with. (LeDoux, 2003). Every thought or emotion that we experience causes a reaction in a specific area of our brain. If our brain recognizes a similarity between a stressful situation from the past with what it hears or sees at the moment, even though there is no current threat or danger, the same distress signals that were experienced in that earlier situation can become activated (Feinstein, 2005). The major conclusion from studies of fear and other emotional conditioning is that the amygdala plays a critical role in linking external stimuli to defense responses. We have the ability to control and modulate instinctive emotional reactions through intellectual processes, such as reasoning, rationalizing, and labeling our experiences. A brain study from UCLA used functional MRI to identify the neural networks underlying this ability. Matching angry or frightened expressions was associated with increased regional cerebral blood flow in the left and right amygdala, the brain's primary fear centers. Labeling these same expressions was associated with a diminished regional cerebral blood flow response in the amygdalae. This decrease correlated with a simultaneous increase in regional cerebral blood flow in the right prefrontal cortex, a neocortical region implicated in regulating emotional responses. These results provide evidence for a network in which higher regions attenuate emotional responses at the most fundamental levels in the brain and suggest a neural basis for controlling emotional experience through interpretation and labeling (Hariri, 2000).

Onion of negative emotions to peel off for better health

According to Gymind, five "negative" emotions: anger, sadness, fear, mental pain and guilt, form an "onion of emotions" that we must all peel off in order to release negativity and let go of mental boundaries that block our way and prevent us from fulfilling everything we wish and ask for in life. If the emotion is negative, then some equivalent biochemical materials are released by the body and may start to accumulate in the body. On an unconscious level, and sometimes consciously, an emotion like anger serves a purpose for u , offering a sense of control maybe, of strength or assertiveness. We think that fear provides us with protection; we presume that guilt may keep us safe from remaking the same mistake. In fact, those emotions don't protect, they reject. They reject goodness and joy; they might "poison" our heart or our mind by guiding energy in the wrong direction. They are "limiting emotions" that limit our freedom, happiness, and health. Guilt energies are some of the heaviest energies to deal with. We observe them as destroying one's self worth and crushing one's purpose in life (Nirula, 1997). Time Line Therapy may very well help us let go of the "root cause" of the negative emotion, hence create a magical shift in our mind and soul, as we have seen earlier in this chapter. Letting go of anger, for instance, doesn't mean never being angry any more. It means that the intensity of anger, experienced before, is no longer there. Anger becomes more deductive or focused, relevant for the case without all the subconscious emotional baggage.

Irene loves the beach, naming it her "therapeutic environment". For years she could not take her three boys with her, relax or enjoy herself at the beach. She was literally hysterical, anxious, shouting, not allowing her three energetic boys to get near the waves without them holding her hands. She was constantly nervous and stressed. Peeling off negative emotions made all that experience much more cheerful. Indeed, Irene still needed to hold her kids' hands near the waves, but her heart was at ease with that and messages such as "the ocean can be a dangerous environment" were delivered peacefully. The boys grasped the message much better when it was delivered firmly yet quietly.

Releasing Anxiety

Anxiety is a feeling of fear, worry, and uneasiness, usually generalized and unfocused as an overreaction to a situation that is only subjectively seen as menacing (Bouras, 2007). It is the subjectively unpleasant feelings of dread over something unlikely to happen, (Davidson, 2008), as a horrible "script" possesses the mind and won't let go, immediately and harshly influencing the body in the form of restlessness, fatigue, problems in concentration, and muscular tension.

The release of anxiety using timeline techniques is so easy and it is recommended to practice on various occasions. After the fourth or fifth time the subconscious begins to generalize this into a functional pattern (Stevenson, 2007). This means that this mind technique "trains" the subconscious mind to always seek the optimistic outcome instead of seeing the "worst case scenario".

Maya's releasing anxiety

Maya experienced anxieties rather often, especially every time she had to go for a physical checkup. Her mind wandered to the worst nightmare, imagining that the cardiologist observed no improvement in her heart condition and that her kids would be raised without their mother. It's with those horrible thoughts that she experienced palpitations, dizziness, fatigue, and shivering. With this simple timeline technique Maya learned to control those thoughts and to calm herself immediately. After a short while, her anxiety on that matter and on other matters subsided significantly.

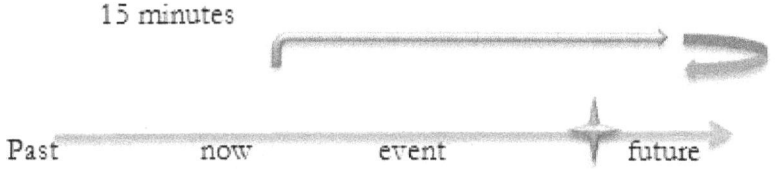

"Float up above your time line and float fifteen minutes past the successful completion of the event about which you thought you were anxious. When you get there, give me a nod".

"Good. Turn around and look toward now on the timeline and ask yourself, now, where is the anxiety? Is it there, or is it gone now"?

As Maya floated 15 minutes past the successful completion of the event, she saw herself after the visit to the cardiologist, calm, reassured, talking on the phone with her husband, about to be reunited with her twins. She instantly smiled, her body became calm and relaxed, and the anxiety was gone.

"Good, go ahead and come back to now over the timeline and come back into the room".

According to Korsybski in his book "Science and Sanity", (1995), all emotions require time to express themselves. This important contribution to timeline techniques was brought by Leslie-Cameron

Bandler and illustrated in the book "Emotional Hostage" in 1986. Switching the perspective on the timeline reframes the emotion into nonexistence. Once the reframe occurs, the emotion loses its context and disappears. In addition to that, according to the book "A Course in Miracles" (1996), there is only one true emotion, that of love. All negative emotions are simply an illusion derived from fear. Switching the temporal perspective shows the negative emotion to be an illusion, and it disappears.

"The cause of all negative emotions is a disruption in the body's energy system": Callahan (1980) and Emotional Freedom Technique

About 5,000 years ago, the Chinese discovered a complex system of energy circuits that run throughout the body. These energy circuits, or Meridians as they are called, are the centerpiece of Eastern health practices and form the basis for modern day acupuncture, acupressure and a wide variety of other healing techniques.

EFT, or Emotional Freedom Technique, is an emotional version of acupuncture except we don't use needles. We do use a simple two-pronged process wherein we mentally "tune in" to specific issues while stimulating certain meridian points on the body by tapping on them with our fingertips. The energy courses through the body, yet is invisible to the eye. By analogy, we do not see the energy flowing through a TV set either. We know it is there - by its effects. In the same way, EFT gives striking evidence that unique energy flows within our meridians because it provides the effects that let us know it is there. By simply tapping near the end points of our energy meridians, we can experience some profound changes in our emotional and physical health. That's what EFT is all about. Western medical science tends to focus on the chemical nature of the body and until recent years, had not paid much attention to these subtle, yet powerful, energy flows. However, they do exist and are attracting an growing group of researchers. For instance, a recent study published in Psychiatry states that "Depression symptoms improve after successful weight loss with Emotional Freedom Techniques" (Stapleton, 2013). A study from the Foundation for Epigenetic Medicine in California praises the effect of EFT on stress biochemistry. This study examined the changes in cortisol levels and psychological distress symptoms of 83 nonclinical subjects receiving a single hour-long intervention, and the results were very clear in favor of the EFT treatment as far as a significant reduction in cortisol levels and psychological stress (Church, 2012). Dr. Feinstein (2012), a clinical psychologist, is an internationally recognized leader in the rapidly emerging field of Energy Psychology. A literature search identified 51 peer-reviewed papers that report or investigate clinical outcomes following the tapping of acupuncture points to address psychological issues. In EFT therapy we do not say that the negative emotion is caused by the memory of the past traumatic experience. The connection of traumatic memories to negative emotions is a mainstay in conventional psychotherapy. EFT, by contrast, respects the memory but addresses the true cause, a disruption in the body's energy system (Callahan, 1985). Properly done, EFT appears to balance disturbances in the meridian system, and thus often reduces the conventional therapy procedures from months or years down to minutes or hours. The basic method presented here is very portable and learnable.

EFT in action

In 1980 Dr. Roger Callahan discovered EFT while working with a patient. In the early 1990s, a Stanford-trained engineer named Gary Craig simplified Callahan's earlier energy psychology (Callahan, 2000). It is practiced with a high degree of uniformity because The EFT Manual, (Craig, 2008), has been available as a free online download since the inception of the method in 1995.

Irene needs to let go of fear.

Stage 1: calibration.

On a scale of one to ten, 1 is lowest and 10 is highest, how frightened are you when your kids go near the waves?

Irene: "8" (expect a quick answer)

Stage 2: The affirmation.

Irene repeats an affirmation 3 times while she rubs the "sore spot" located in the upper left and right portions of the chest, right under the clavicle, where lymphatic congestion occur.

Even though I am afraid when my kids approach the waves, I deeply and completely accept myself.

This is how Irene acknowledges the problem and creates self-acceptance despite the existence of the problem. That is what's necessary for the affirmation to be effective.

Stage 3: The sequence.

It's time to tap on the end points of the major energy meridians, usually more convenient to practice with the dominant hand, index finger and middle finger joined together to cover larger area. Tap a few times on each of the tapping points (Graig, 2012).

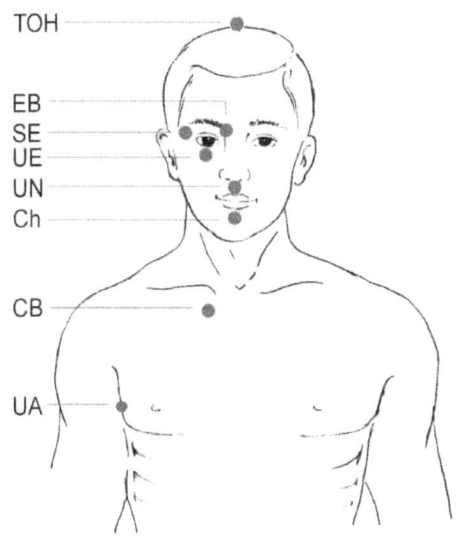

TOH
EB
SE
UE
UN
Ch
CB
UA

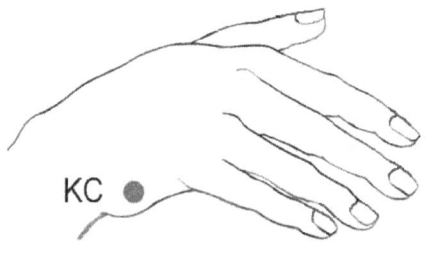

KC

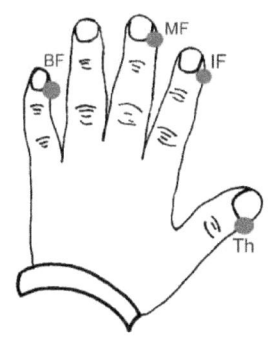

MF
BF
IF
Th

TOH: On the top of the head. If you were to draw a line from one ear, over the head, to the other ear and another line from your nose to the back of your neck, the TOH point is where those two lines would intersect.

EB: At the beginning of the eyebrow, just above and to one side of the nose. This point is abbreviated EB for beginning of the EyeBrow.

SE: On the bone bordering the outside corner of the eye. This point is abbreviated SE for Side of the Eye.

UE: On the bone under an eye about 1 inch below your pupil. This point is abbreviated UE for Under the Eye.

UN: On the small area between the bottom of your nose and the top of your upper lip. This point is abbreviated UN for Under the Nose.

Ch: Midway between the point of your chin and the bottom of your lower lip. Even though it is not directly on the point of the chin, we call it the chin point because it is descriptive enough for people to understand easily. This point is abbreviated Ch for Chin.

CB: The junction where the sternum (breastbone), collarbone, and the first rib meet. To locate it, first place your forefinger on the U-shaped notch at the top of the breastbone (about where a man would knot his tie). From the bottom of the U, move your forefinger down toward the navel 1 inch and then go to the left (or right) 1 inch. This point is abbreviated CB for Collarbone even though it is not on the collarbone (or clavicle) per se.

UA: On the side of the body, at a point even with the nipple (for men) or in the middle of the bra strap (for women).

KC: The Karate Chop point (abbreviated KC) is located at the center of the fleshy part of the outside of your hand (either hand) between the top of the wrist and the base of the baby finger. This is the part of your hand you would use to deliver a karate chop.

The Finger Points: The tapping point is in the same location for each finger and each thumb. On the index finger (IF), tap on the side of the finger that is closest to the thumb, even with the base of the nail. Once you have located that one, you can find the similar MF (middle finger), BF (baby finger), and Th (thumb) points on each hand. The Ring Finger has not been included in this sequence, since the meridian involved runs on the opposite side of that finger.

Stage 4: "Fine tune" the brain with the gamut procedure.

Through connecting nerves, certain parts of the brain are stimulated when the eyes are moved. It's also the right side of the brain, the creative side, engaged when we hum a song, and the left side, the digital side, engaged when we count.

Eyes closed.

Eyes open.

Eyes hard down right while holding the head steady.

Eyes hard down left while holding the head steady.

Roll your eyes in a circle as though your nose was at the center of a clock, and you were trying to see all the numbers in order.

Same as #5, only reverse the direction in which you roll your eyes.

Hum 2 seconds of a song (any song will do).

Count rapidly from 1 to 5.

Hum 2 seconds of a song again.

Stage 5: Repeat stage 3, the sequence.

Stage 6: calibration.

Irene rerates the intensity of the trauma on the 1 to 10 scale. If the number is still high, (let's say 6), EFT is applied again, stages 1-6.

EFT and children

EFT can do wonders with children. They often feel ticklish, they laugh a lot, they enjoy the process of tapping. Their lack of skepticism, their ability to devote themselves to the process, and their connection to originality and nature – all these enable them to be open to the EFT process and to any healing process, for that matter. Children are without any "masks", they are pure, willing, and attentive, especially to their inner voice, their intuition, and their mental and emotional needs.

Oliver's inner world

We remember Oliver's wonderful progress. From a hypotonic, overweight, and somewhat socially challenged kid, Oliver's striving for a change in life was admirable and inspiring. Along with fitness and proper nutrition, Oliver devoted himself completely to the mental emotional and spiritual part of his life. The way to "reach" Oliver for the first encounters was not obvious. EFT was a wonderful "ice breaker" in the first two sessions. It was for him a practical and fun tool, bizarre and unique with no need for Oliver to speak and verbally share his feelings. Oliver's affirmation was "Even though I am somewhat overweight, I deeply and completely accept myself". He seemed to fully understand this affirmation, the fact that only by acceptance of the problem, are we able to solve it and release it. Calibration was challenging in this case since we could not calibrate Oliver's physical situation from a scale of 1 to 10. However, we could sense how much tapping really made him feel better about himself. Two rounds of EFT made it possible for us to concentrate on other aspects, and Oliver's whole transformation became easier thanks to the emotional tools we used.

As an infant, Oliver's speech was constructed by associations. His mom revealed that he had a habit of talking to his hands as if they were puppets, making his inner worlds "blend" with reality. It's that same magical quality Oliver possessed that helped him later at the age of 12 get reconnected to his profound and rich inner world. Oliver has a tempestuous and stormy spirit that characterizes artists and philosophers. This was not hard to notice right from the start. His mind wondered occasionally to deep thoughts and really smart questions about Greek mythology or "Dungeons and Dragons"; conversations about death and where the spirit wanders off when it leaves the body. Fearless, yet a deep thinker, sessions with Oliver were emotional, spiritual and apparently essential to help this wonderful kid fit into the world. EFT and Time Line therapy enabled Oliver to reunite with the inner voice he had to moderate as an infant in order to fit into the "outer" world. Later on, when Oliver turned 14 and Theta-Healing therapy was added to the Gymind treasure chest of tools, Oliver got some more answers to his everlasting spiritual questions.

The sixth sense and our health: More than meets the eye

Even though we live in the golden era of brain research, as Chopra puts it (2012), the study of the mind remains limited. One of the most influential and inspiring movies on that subject was released in 2011: _Limitless_, an American mystery thriller film directed by Neil Burger and starring Bradley Cooper, Abbie Cornish, and Robert De Niro.[8] With the help of a mysterious pill that enables the user to access 100 percent of his brain abilities, Eddie, the main character, finds that he is able to learn faster and recall memories from his distant past and predict the future. His mind is sharper than ever, and he possesses the key to endless opportunities. It's a movie of "what

---

8 _Limitless_ is based on the 2001 novel The Dark Fields by Alan Glynn with the screenplay by Leslie Dixon.

ifs": What if we were able to use all 100 percent of our brain, what if we had the key to endless opportunities. Humanity is not there yet. Even the greatest brain surgeons and the best neurologists remain in the dark as far as the endless capacities of the brain and endless possibilities it holds within. It's not only the "brain doctors", but western medicine as a whole. Certainly, we all benefit from conventional medicine. Far beyond medications and progress, the essence of conventional medicine has its own powerful spiritual vibration and it is up to us to use it wisely. But our body consists of more than just matter, or cells running around with automatic responses communicating with each other like a "biological machine". Feelings, emotions, beliefs - they all influence how we behave and have dramatic effects on the body's well-being, even at the cellular level. The cells, in the brain and in the body as a whole, are very aware of the environment both inside and outside the body and have individual intelligence, while still remaining connected to the whole (Stibal, 2008). Far beyond what "meets the eye", along with smell, touch, hear, taste – there is this certain "je ne sais quoi", this certain "energy" we have to consider when we strive for happiness, self-fulfillment, abundance, and health. I once heard a phrase that I tend to use often: "A dark room is not necessarily emptied of furniture". While once radio waves seemed atopic we now may not be so surprised that we think of someone and he suddenly calls. Thoughts are those "radio waves", feelings and emotions from our "energetic DNA" that determine our reality for better or for worse, depending on us. We may be born with a certain biological DNA but we also possess this energetic DNA that we should recognize first, and then alter, if we choose to.

The way Gymind utilizes that "sixth sense" varies dramatically from one individual to another. Some are very much open to the spiritual side of the process, captivated by its wonders; some are more careful, attentive only in due time, convinced gradually; some remain skeptical, cynical, or simply "not interested". Through fitness and Nutrition their body can make a tremendous shift for the best. But when people are really open to spirituality - wonders occur. We have experienced that with NLP, Time Line, and EFT. Where NLP addresses the subject of how to "run our own brain" so that we can take charge of the cognitive-behavioral mechanisms that control subjectivity (Bodenhamer, 1998), the "sixth sense" takes us "higher" than that to what Stibal refers to as "the creator of all that is". When we let go of three important components: fear, skepticism and lack of belief, we are opened to turn the light on in that dark room and clean up the room. Meditation, Guided Imagination, Relaxation, Theta-Healing, a healing touch, they may all help us do just that. The word "heal" comes from the same root, meaning "whole, complete" meaning "integrated" and also "holy". The human body is holy (oxymoron? Maybe not), and is strongly connected with its internal health-maintaining intelligence. No matter which method is used for healing, the healer is actually within, not outside. No physician has ever healed anyone. At best he can create conditions where the internal healer gets the best possible conditions to do the healing work (Nirula, 1997).

Circles of energy: Colorful chakras for constancy and balance

In the Journal of Holistic Nursing, Slater (1995) discusses the human electromagnetic characteristics, compared to descriptions of auras, meridians, and chakras. Quantum and chaos theories are presented and applied to the question of the mechanism of energetic healing. Chakras are a system of subtle energy bodies or vortexes or wheels on the body which act like energy transformers. From Sanskrit: 'wheel', spinning vortex of energy in the human energy field (aura) that works as energy accumulators and pumps (Nirual, 1997). In Chapter One we discussed the lower chakra and the importance of walking or running for health, security, and dynamic presence. Earlier in this chapter we encountered with the "third eye" chakra in the hakalau vision.

Many of the problems that we experience in day-to-day life can be attributed to imbalance in one of the main chakras. When our chakras are out of balance or blocked, it will disrupt our entire physical system, eventually result in mental, emotional or physical illness. (Rose, 2013). We need to cleanse and balance our chakras constantly to maintain a balance of energy. By removing such blockages and maximizing energy flow, it enables the body, mind and spirit to function optimally. Chakras are checked by working off the body and feeling the etheric field around them, or by using pendulum and muscle testing. Every session is different and how chakras get balanced will be different for every individual and their needs. Color, sound, energy, and physical work are used in chakra balancing.

1. Base of Spine: Red: Earth, physical identity, oriented to self-preservation. Located at the base of the spine, this chakra forms our foundation. It represents the element of earth, and is therefore related to our survival instincts.

2. Abdomen Chakra: Orange: The second chakra, located in the abdomen, lower back and sexual organs, is related to the element water and to emotions and sexuality. It connects us to others through feeling, desire, sensation, and movement. Ideally this chakra brings us fluidity and grace, depth of feeling, sexual fulfillment, and the ability to accept change.

3. Solar Plexus, the third chakra: Yellow. This chakra is known as the power chakra, located in the solar plexus. It rules our personal power, will and autonomy, as well as our metabolism.

4. Heart Chakra: Green: This chakra is called the heart chakra and is the middle chakra in a system of seven. A healthy fourth chakra allows us to love deeply, feel compassion, and have a deep sense of peace and centeredness.

5. Throat Chakra: blue: throat sound, creative identity, oriented to self-expression, this is the chakra located in the throat and is thus related to communication and creativity.

6. Third Eye Chakra: Purple: Activated in a hakalau vision for example, this chakra is known as the brow chakra or third eye center. It is related to the act of seeing, both physically and intuitively, allowing us to see clearly, letting us "see the big picture."

7. Crown Chakra: White: thought, universal identity, oriented to self-knowledge, this is the crown chakra that relates to consciousness as pure awareness. It is our connection to the greater world beyond, to a timeless place of all-knowing. When developed, this chakra brings us knowledge, wisdom, understanding and spiritual connection.

Matt is balancing his Chakras

Almost two years ago, Matt the pediatrician, 48, whom we met in Chapter Two, was diagnosed with a fatal kind of throat cancer. Since Matt practices medicine, he noticed at a very early stage that something was wrong, and he was diagnosed early enough. PET-CT scans for the past year and a half have been showing his complete recovery. We don't really know why Matt got cancer. It may be irrelevant now that his is healthy. Yet Matt, was gradually "convinced" over the years that Gymind doesn't need to be only about fitness and nutrition, and is a very "intuitive" doctor himself, compassionate, understanding and rooting for the mind as a powerful tool for healing, so he was willing to cooperate. He confessed that pressure and stress play a big part in his life. He rarely takes a deep breath and even though he lacks for nothing financially, he does worry a lot about money and financial security for his family. Matt feels pressure when he is not communicating his emotions and his worries properly. Living with a shopaholic wife makes that kind of communication challenging. Fitness helps a lot to ease that pressure, but apparently it is not enough. Ever since his recovery we balance his chakras almost every session, mainly when Matt asks for it, when life is too stressful to handle. After 50 minutes of physical training Matt lies down comfortably, palms of his hands facing up for a "receiving-energy-position", he takes three deep breaths and devotes himself to acceptance, good energy, and flow. We sometimes use energetic crystals based on each chakra, and sometimes simply the energy of my palms combined with some guided imagination will suffice.

Mediation for balanced chakras

Sit back and relax in a chair that supports your back and your body comfortably. Close your eyes. Bring your attention to your breathing, without trying to change it. Just observe it as you breathe in and out for a few minutes. (Well-Being Alignment, LLC, 2013). Then you can read a section at a time, close your eyes to do each step, or you can record the meditation and listen to it in your own voice.

Imagine this stream of pure White Light Healing Energy flows down from above your head and into the top of your head, a glorious waterfall of pure white, just like water coming from above, caressing your body. Only this light enters your body, and when it flows down, it feels unconditional love, wellbeing, vitality and joy, straight from above, from the heart of the Creator, flowing into your being. This pure white light healing energy shines like millions of diamonds, reflecting all the colors of the rainbow, each color carrying a specific ray of healing and nourishment into all levels of your Being. Your body knows exactly which color it needs, and every cell is enlightened and nurtured.

You breathe in this white light healing energy all the way down to the soles of your feet, out your feet and deep into the core of Mother Earth. You are creating a permanent, continuous corridor of light from the Heart of Source, from the creation above, down through all levels of your being and deep into beloved Mother Earth. As your breath goes out, you breathe this white light healing energy out from your heart to all humanity.

From your Crown Chakra you breathe this pure diamond light into the middle of your forehead, into your third eye. You release everything that has blocked your reception of the Highest Light and Love of Source. Ask this white light healing energy to open your inner vision to a broader, light-filled, continually expanding perspective. From the top of your head, you breathe the pure healing light and Love of Source into your Throat, your place of speaking and being your Truth. You release everything that veils the Truth of Who you are. As you breathe out, the pure white light healing energy from above your being flows through your throat and out to all humanity, bringing light, healing, and love to the world through your voice.

Still breathing in white diamond light into the crown of your head, you breathe it down into your Heart Chakra, expanding your heart in a brilliant sphere of pure white light, radiating out in all directions. In this light healing, you release everything that has veiled love. You breathe out white light healing energy to all humanity through your heart center.

From your Crown Chakra you breathe in the pure white light healing energy into your solar plexus, just below your heart. You are an expanding unified field of pure white light as you breathe healing light into, within, through and around your body.

As you continue breathing in pure white light healing energy from the crown of your head down, you breathe it into your sacral chakra just below your navel. You feel joy as pure white healing light, unconditional love and divine compassion nurture this joy, surrender everything that veils light. You are a unified field of pure white light, and breathe healing light and wellbeing into, within, though, and around your body.

From the top of your head, you breathe in pure white light healing energy down into your root chakra at the base of your spine, feeling your tribal connection with Mother Earth and all your fellow human beings. You release all separating and constricting imprints stored in your root chakra. You are a unified field of pure white light, breathing healing light into, within, through and around your body.

With each breath, this healing light expands out in a brilliant sphere of white light all around your physical body. You are a unified field of pure, brilliant white light, within, through and around your body. Through your heart center I breathe out this brilliant healing light to all humanity. You accept this white light healing, Beloved you are.

Take a deep breath and open your eyes (wellbeingalignment.com).

Seven planes of existence

In order to fully grasp this "spiritual healing" and maintenance of mental balance and healthy mindset, it is important to explore this model of planes we live in. Health can be attained in many ways according to that model, and it will gradually bring us up into the seventh plane, to the Creator of all, that is, the energy of creation, ultimate joy, abundance, and healing. It is important to understand these seven planes in order to clarify why and where our beliefs, programs, contracts, commitments, initiations and healings originate. We operate physically, emotionally, mentally and spiritually, connected to all planes and being a part of them. Every plane works in our body in complete harmony to create life at all times. Every plane operates within this third plane, the "Now", where we, as humans, reside. Since we utilize and work with these planes both consciously and unconsciously, it is essential that we learn to respect the awareness that these planes bring forth (Ben-Israel, 2012).

The First Plane of Existence is where molecules come together to form non-carbon based matter. This is the power of Mother Earth. Examples of the 1st plane elements are rocks, minerals, and earth. Taking mineral supplements such as calcium and magnesium are provided from this plane and give support to our physical bodies. The crystals we might use when balancing Matt's chakras come from the first plane of existence.

The Second Plane of Existence is the first time the molecules merge with carbon. This plane includes organic matter: plants, herbs, trees, vitamins, viruses, bacteria, mold, yeast and fungus. A sacred dance is created between the plant beings along with the Earth/Air Spirits to interconnect between the first and third plane of existence. Water resonates at this level as well.

The Third Plane of Existence is an illusion, the reality being what we, as humans, create in it. It is a playground on which to work with emotions, passion, and creativity. It is a place to learn to control our thoughts and master our fears, as fear is the only thing that keeps us thinking that we are bound to this illusion and separate from the seventh plane and the "creator of all that is". The more beliefs we change, the faster we can shift through all the planes freely, no longer bond by Karma, (the law of cause and effect from the 6th Plane). Animals also exist in this plane.

Between the third and fourth plane is where wayward (discarnate spirits) get "stuck" between the Earth and the electromagnetic grid or energy (it is again, part of the laws of the universe in the 6th plane).

The Fourth Plane of Existence is where totems, (animal spirits), shape shifters and many ancestors' spirits reside. People who work constantly on this plane are called shamans. It is the plane where the soul waits to take form again (reincarnate) and genetic beliefs get passed on. Language originates from the fourth plane and is used by third plane inhabitants. There was a time when we once could hear and see all, we would just "know" without the use of language.

When Tami, a 12-year-old girl, confided in me that she sometime cannot resist a chocolate bar and that she experiences some major difficulties in restraining herself from social eating with friends, hence raising her daily calorie consumption higher than recommended. I suggested we find her a Totem-Animal to help and guide her through those difficult times. So we went for a meditative journey to find and get reconnected to Tami's Spirit Animal. "Take three deep breaths and close your eyes. Imagine you are in the woods; I can join you if you need me to, so you can hold my hand. We are walking in the woods, the sky is blue, birds are singing, our bare feet touch the soft ground and with every step we take you feel reconnected to mother earth. In a minute we will see these stairs that lead us deep down into the ground. The stairs are inviting, wide and comfortable. Curious, we take several steps down into the beautiful ground into this large illuminated cave. You take a sit next to this wooden table and you wait for your totem animal to appear before you. The sound of drums plays in the background and you patiently wait. Some animals may appear before you. But once your totem animal is there, you will instantly recognize it. Let's take a few minutes for you to get in touch with it".

Tami did not hesitate and very quickly recognized her animal, a dolphin. I guided Tami to talk to her animal, to ask it to join her whenever she needed it, to protect her, to guide her especially when Tami is facing difficulties with her diet. I asked Tami if the dolphin answered back. She nodded. "What does it say?" "The dolphin agrees with me, it will come to my reality with me. It asks me to swim freely and go with my natural feelings. It will help me do that in my world".

The Fifth Plane of Existence is the astral plane based in dualism, of both love and fear, good and evil. It is a divided realm with a clear separation between the "Upper" and "Lower" aspects of this plane. There are the high vibratory energies who live at the "upper spectrum" like the higher self, gods, goddesses, guardian angels, legions of celestial angels, master angels, guides, Christ, Buddha, Jehovah, Yahweh, Heavenly Mother and Father and the Councils of 12 (heads of soul family gatherings). Then there are the "lower" 5th plane realms of the fallen angels[9], demons, Satan. These divisions do not intermingle among each other though they are very aware of their

---

9 A fallen angel is a wicked or rebellious angel that has been cast out of heaven. The term is found neither in the Hebrew Bible nor the Deuterocanonical Books nor the New Testament. Nonetheless, Biblical commentators often use 'fallen angel' to describe angels who sinned or angels cast down to the earth from the war in heaven. (Bamberger, 2006).

existences.

The Sixth Plane of Existence is the plane of laws of creation. There are billions of laws some of which are Light (color), Sound (tone), Karma, (cause and effect), Attraction, Justice, Wisdom, Balance, Gravity, Magnetics, and Electricity. This plane also includes the formation and awareness of numbers, which can be expressed as patterns and symbols (astrology and numerology). This is where the laws of the subconscious mind reside. Under the law of time are actually dimensions, sacred geometry. There is no Law of Love, as love just IS.

The Seventh Plane of Existence is where pure love and the highest true reside. It is the plane of the creator of all that is, ALL of creation creates all the other planes as IT exists throughout everything. In the seventh plane resides the pure energy of the creation that gives security, change of energy for the best and instant pure healing. This plane simply holds and caresses unconditionally and effortlessly while being able to use all the other planes for perfect manifestations, without rules, boundaries or conditions. We can all rejoin and utilize this plane, since we use our inhibited right to be a part of "all that is" without any separations. Going to the seventh plane eliminates ego and sickness; allows us to witness healings; allows us to know the highest truth; aligns us to travel to any plane so that we can move between the planes with consciousness and communicate with physical elements and stops us from being committed or obligated to the laws or rules of other planes of existence. The more people who tap into the Group Collective Consciousness to witness change at this seventh plane, the easier it will be to shift human consciousness. We can evolve together and have instantaneous healings all the time (www.thetadnaactivation.com).

Vianna Stibal's revelation: Theta-Healing
In Theta-Healing we have been given a meditation that allows us to 'remember' our connection to this All-That-Is-Creation, as there is no

possible way we were or have ever been disconnected from IT. Theta-Healing is designed to open up our psychic abilities to heal. In the 1990s in Idaho, Vianna Stibal stumbled upon a remarkable discovery. Not only did she have the natural gift to "read" inside people's bodies with great accuracy, but she could also witness their healings unfolding right in front of her inner eye. She herself was diagnosed with a malignant tumor in her right leg, and a biopsy left her with excruciating pain and on crutches for six weeks but she continued to give massages and intuitive readings to people, certain that the Creator of All There Is could heal her in an instant. And so IT did. Stibal tells how one day while limping down the street, it occurred to her that if she could witness others heal, maybe she could also heal herself and in that moment God responded to her affirmation, and her leg returned to its normal length. Stibal did not exactly know at the time why the healing occurred but after doing some thorough research, she concluded that she must be slowing her brain waves to theta while witnessing the healing which allows the healing to solidify most effectively. She began to teach this method to anyone who cared to listen and named it "Theta Healing".

Theta and other brain waves

The human brain produces different levels of electrical activity depending on the amount of information it is processing. During a detailed task, it lights up with electrical charges as it sends and receives messages in high concentration, its neurons fire in quick succession. While the person is in a relaxed state of sleep, its neurons fire less often. This brainwave activity is calculated by electroencephalographs, (EEGs), machines that gather data from electrodes affixed to the skull and measure the amount of electric activity per unit of time, (frequency), in Hertz. (Inman, 2011).

Throughout the day, the brain ranges between four different types of brainwave patterns:

Beta (12 -30 Hz), the normal, wakeful consciousness associated with activity.

Alpha (8 – 12 Hz), the relaxed and reflective state, like that induced by closing the eyes during waking hours.

Theta (4 – 7 Hz), a very relaxed state associated with meditation, hypnosis, lucid dreaming, and the barely conscious state just before sleeping and just after waking. Theta is the border between the conscious and the subconscious world; by learning to use conscious, waking Theta brain waves, we can access and influence the powerful subconscious part of ourselves that is normally inaccessible to our waking minds. While in the Theta state, the mind is capable of deep and profound learning, healing, and growth. (Brent, 2012).

Delta, (3 and under Hz), deep, dreamless sleep.

A study from the Veterans Administration Medical Center in Colorado found alpha-theta brainwave biofeedback training most effective as a novel treatment technique for chronic alcoholics. Application of brainwave treatment, a relaxation therapy, appears to counteract the increase in circulating beta-endorphin levels seen in the control group of alcoholics (Peniston, 1989). Theta waves allow a person to experience extreme relaxation, creativity, as well as vibrant mental imagery. Our brain slows down to this frequency under several different circumstances, all of which allow us to access greater creativity and for lack of a better word, a more "elastic" reality. It grants us the possibility to experience reality more vividly, more multi-dimensionally. During the moments between waking and sleep, we can somehow experience a reality independent of physical laws, free of earth-bound conditioning. For a moment, even though we are already awake, limited by our sensory perception, we can still sense a different reality where we possess almost super human powers, just as in "Limitless". With the help of these brainwaves, the intuitive capacity increases, the ability to "see" and to "hear" outside the boundaries of the physical senses expands, and we can shift our limited perception of reality (Golan, 2012). Everyone can do it. We train our brains to awaken a latent ability and direct our senses to believe in unlimited possibilities. All we need is a belief in a higher power and a desire to find and express our fullest capacity as human beings. We must strive for more; believe that we have powers greater than what science, medicine, or any other authority claims we have. The more we exercise our multi-dimensional vision of reality, the more we can express a higher potential for humanity. Stibal understood that healing was one of the theta brainwave's functions. According to her revelation, once she projected her consciousness above her space and called upon the Creator, her brainwaves slowed down to a theta state in less than 30 seconds and she then was able to witness miraculous things happen. The Creator was doing the healing but she had to witness it in order for it to manifest in the physical dimension. Until it is witnessed, it remains in the realm of potentiality. Once we can "see" the healing unfold and "know" that it is "done", it can happen. In the 4-7 cycles per second frequency, the mind is able to access limitless possibilities outside the realm of the sensory perception.

Entering the seventh plane

This meditation is a direct reading from the book "Theta Healing" by Stibal. It is used as a "road map" to the "seventh plane" to enter the theta brain wave state and connect with Creator Consciousness. We can use this for entering a state to create healing or manifestation. For the most part, just the basic healing, just going to the Creator of All that Is and commanding the body to heal can do amazing things (Stibal, 2008).

Imagine energy coming up from the center of the earth, going all the way up to the bottom of your feet, this energy is drawn up through all of your chakra's centers and comes up out of the top of your head as a beautiful ball of light. Your consciousness is in this ball of light. Take time to notice what color it is. Now imagine going up above your space, above this room, above the building, further up into the sky, further up above the earth, higher, above the galaxy, all the way up above the universe, you see a light above the universe it is a big beautiful light, imagine going up through that light and you see another bright light and another and another…there are many bright lights. Keep going. Keep going all the way up. Finally there is a great big bright light. Go through it and when you go through it, you see this energy that is a gel-like substance that has all the colors of the rainbow in it. When you go into it, you see that it changes colors. This is the Laws. You will see all kinds of shapes and colors. In the distance that is a white light, it is a bright blue color like a pearl. Head for that light, as you get closer you see a mist of pink; keep going. This is the law of compassion and it will push you into the special place. You will see that the light is like a window, this window is the opening to the seventh plane. Now go through it, go deep within it. See a deep brightish glow that goes through your body dissolving the ball of energy surrounding you, you feel it going through your body, it feels light but it has essence. You feel it going through you as you no longer feel the separation between your own body and the energy. You become all that is. Your body will not disappear; it will become perfect and healthy. There is nothing but energy here. It is from this place that the Creator of all that is can do healings that will heal instantly, and it is from this place that you can create in all aspects of your life. You dissolve into the love of the creator of all that is, there is no fear, you just gently feel this energy moving through everything, you realize that you are a part of everything and everyone. It is easy to manifest in this energy because you realize that you are part of everybody and everything that is. You can feel the energy all around you as you realize your body has come into perfect balance. Now is the time to think about what it is that you want in your life. Imagine that it is sitting in your life already and that you are a part of it. Take a deep breath in, open your eyes feeling totally connected to all that is. It is from this place that you get connected to all that is, and it is from this place that you can change the outcome and energy in your life.

Rainbow children and theta-healing

Rainbow Children are incredibly sensitive intuitive children, teens and adults. A rainbow child is a child born with unlimited intelligence and the ability to change the energy around him (Weaver, 2013). Since the beginning of time, the world has waited for these tremendously loving and adaptable rainbow children to come in with their unlimited love and tolerance. Intuitively they are connected to the seventh plane of existence, totally connected to the creator of all that is, brilliant, creative, psychic, and manifesters. Whatever they need or desire, they can instantly manifest (Brown, 2013). Rainbow children bring joy and harmony to their families. Born to smile, with huge hearts that are full of forgiveness, the rainbow child generally recovers from the state of negative emotion quickly. At a young age, the rainbow children are able to express their needs and wants. These children actually own a great deal of personal power. Rainbow children may be misinterpreted as stubborn.

Doreen Virtue, known as "The Angel Lady"[10] says that the rainbow children are perfectly balanced in their male and female energies, meaning they are confident without aggressiveness; they are intuitive and psychic without effort; they are magical and can bend time, become invisible and go without sleep and food. The rainbow children operate purely out of joy, not out of need or impulse. Parents will realize that they cannot out-give their rainbow children, for these children are a mirror of all actions and energy of love. These children will play an important role in the earth's evolution. They have healing abilities and telepathy. (Pattillo, 2007). They heal

10 Doreen Virtue holds B.A., M.A., and Ph.D. degrees in counseling psychology; she is a lifelong clairvoyant who works with the angelic realm. She is the author of "Assertiveness for Earth Angels," "The Miracles of Archangel Gabriel," and many decks of angel oracle cards, among other works. Doreen has appeared on Oprah, The View, Good Morning America, CNN, and other programs and presents workshops around the world; she also has a weekly call-in talk show on hayhouseradio.com.

us with their huge heart chakras.

The Children's Castle meditation for love and manifestation

Take a deep breath and close your eyes. Imagine you are at the beach, looking at the blue sea, walking on the white sand, feeling the sand caressing your feet, smelling the wonderful smell of the sea, hearing the seagulls, watching them play above your head. You feel joy and happiness. As you continue to walk along the beach, you spot a beautiful crystal castle far at the horizon. You gradually approach that magnificent colorful castle as you see your name on the gate. You gently open the gate and you enter this wide, long bright corridor. As you start to walk through that corridor, you see that the walls are actually mirrors. And you see yourself first as a baby, then as an infant, getting bigger and taller until you see yourself as you appear today and you reach the end of the corridor. As you reach the end of that corridor, you hear people calling your name. You approach those people only to realize that those are angels: beautiful, gentle, colorful, bright angels. And they hug you, telling you how wonderful you are, how much you are wanted and loved. How much joy you bring with you to the world and how powerful your being is. They escort you into this light, a wonderful bright light. And as you gently enter that light, that energy of all that is, you know it has EVERYTHING in it, even-though it seems empty. You take a deep breath; you feel that bright white endless energy caressing your body. You can ask for ANYTHING you want, feeling how much EVERYTHING is possible. And you stay in the white bright light until you witness how your wish is fulfilled. You then rejoin the angels. They escort you into that corridor of mirrors into the beautiful beach and as you feel the warm wind on your face and as you hear the singing of the seagulls, you can open your eyes and come back into the room.

Not yet the end: Know yourself, take charge and set a goal to manifest health and abundance

Who really knows what secrets lie in the depth of the brain? It may take years and years of neurological research to find out, and we are not quite there yet. For now, we can and should focus on what we do know and choose to "be at cause", knowing, according to Hermann Hesse's famous quote, that "There is no reality except the one contained within us. That is why so many people live such an unreal life. They take the images outside of them for reality and never allow the world within to assert itself."

Irene, Emma, Matt, Belle, Barak, Oliver, Tami, Ave, Maya, Aida, they all stopped blaming reality, life, others and chose to take charge over their own course of action, over their emotions, thoughts, and dreams. Irene defies the "laws of Lupus" which weaken her body, and she overcomes and controls her fears by using the Emotional Freedom Technique therapy. Emma is finally "driving the bus", holding the steering wheel and navigating her way with the right mindset. Both Belle and Aida took the time to face the past and with the help of a resourced anchor and guided imagination, let go of images that had been stored in their mind since childhood, blocking the way for a better future. Barak embraced physiology of excellence to gain professional and personal confidence; he learned all about his and his wife's representational systems for better communication, understanding and peace of mind. Oliver and Tami, both "rainbow children" got reconnected to this powerful "seventh place of existence" a la Theta Healing where the energy of "all that is" fulfills them and enables them to meet with their endless abilities. Ave uses her "third eye" and her strong intuition for controlling her eating habits. Maya got connected to her timeline in order to heal her heart.

The belief and feeling work are designed to change the way we send and receive messages in the body. It's when we replace enough programs in a person's brain so that the right chemical messengers are released and the receptors accept the message as valid, allowing the physical change to miraculously occur. We are all unique individuals with unique needs and personal belief systems, knowing that even if we have the same problem, it does not mean that we can solve it in the same way. Whether we believe that Neuro-linguistic programming is a tool for health, or perhaps the Emotional Freedom Technique, TimeLine Therapy, or the phenomenal Theta Healing therapy, it's up to us to reconnect to our wonderful limitless self and get healthy. We do not have to know all the secrets that lie deep in the brain, but we do need to know that we have a resilient body that we should bless and encourage; that when we believe healing or change in all areas of life is possible, then the body will respond and so will reality.

The brain is constantly evolving, hence we are constantly evolving, choosing the way up through the stairways of life. Taking a higher step may be challenging and hard. We practice every muscle in our thigh, putting all of our weight on that small foot and we make the effort to take that step. It's hard. But when we do that, we are placed in a higher position, looking back to where we came from, being able to see better from above, and having a better perspective on life.

Where are they today?

"A man is but the product of his thoughts. What he thinks, he becomes," so wisely asserted Gandhi, Indian political and spiritual leader (1869 – 1948). Yet thoughts, as vital and significant as they are, represent only a fraction of our being. The strong and uncompromising linkage between Body: Fitness and Nutrition and Mind: Conscious and Subconscious, heart and soul, and by all means, thoughts, embodies the main objective of this book you hold. The first two chapters touch upon the tangible, hence the concrete and corporal: Workouts, physical conceptions, nutrition plans, in hope of proposing a practical and enjoyable physical plan and a wide range of possibilities for more active, colorful, and "tasteful" life. The third chapter touches upon the intangible: Words, thoughts, amygdala, emotions, imagination, soul and spirit, in hope of proposing an improved mindset and some practical-spiritual tools, as contradictory at it may seem. Gymind is all about those "practical- spiritual" tools when "Gymnastics" meets "Mind", and they are put together as a way of life, for a better quality of life. I have had, and with the writing of those lines, I still have the privilege and the honor to escort many wonderful individuals in their path for health. Gymind as a methodology aspires to be the home for all those who wish to take charge and take care of themselves.

As life continues and personal timelines constantly emerge, let us observe the current state of some of those individuals we have encountered along the road:

Maya is happily raising her 20-month-old twins. Her physical condition, as far as cardiovascular abilities, is getting better by the minute, and she is stronger than ever. Maya rarely feels any palpitations, she is much more relaxed now, and anxieties are rapidly becoming a distant memory. When fear takes over or emotional needs increase, she either uses the EFT technique, or she anchors herself to her two precious babies. She is currently contemplating a second career and thinking about becoming a therapist. She feels the urge to help other women who have experienced similar mental and physical difficulties. As for now, active in medical forums and helping her close circle, she is on the verge of finding her "sacred destination" in life.

Matt has been healthy and free of cancer for the past year and a half now. Still maintaining a balanced weight and an active life-style of a busy and well-regarded pediatrician, Matt is more open to spirituality. We often keep the last minutes of the session for relaxation, breathing, and meditation. Matt floats easily over his timeline, releases negative emotions - mainly from his recent encounter with cancer - amazed again and again by the power of his mind as far as imagination, visualization, and the way they physically influence his body. Guided imagination and awareness of breathing have become increasingly present in his life, helping him balance himself and release tensions that often occur.

Oliver has grown into quite a handsome young man, so far from that chubby-feeble-timid 12-year-old of three years ago, taller than his two older brothers, physically stronger and mentally much more confident. We are currently working on his posture. His fast growth and his height make his back bend a little, so that we systematically strengthen his shoulders, back, and core muscles. Oliver is also into basketball and tennis, which he enjoys as an aerobic activity. Surrounded with friends, he is doing great in school. All those memories as a toddler, challenged with accepting the outer-world and possessing a richer inner-world are still part of his being, concealed in his body and mind. No wonder he strives now to be like everybody else, sometimes at the expense of finding his own voice. Now he must select a course at school, and he is struggling inwardly: on the one hand he wishes to go with the flow, be accepted by his friends and hence needs to choose the same course as his friends – biology or math. On the other hand, his inner world and artistic spirit attract him to choose the Arts or Theater. What will he finally choose? This is a "healthy" natural conflict from which Oliver will grow even stronger. Time will tell.

Muriel, for the past four years, has kept her weight off, and we believe that she will stay energetic, vital and thin indefinitely. Always devoted to the Gymind way, Muriel takes everything she knows wherever she goes, even to Australia where she is currently travelling, focusing on her happiness, her confidence, and health. Single for so many years while trying not only to lose the weight and keep it off but also to accept and love herself as a whole, Muriel has found a great guy, and they are planning a future together.

Liana is growing into a strong, beautiful young lady. Now at the age of 6, she enjoys outdoors activities, playing outside with friends, or riding her bike. She is proud to show me how she easily and effortlessly climbs the stairs, placing one foot at a time on the step instead of placing both feet together on the same step as she did back when her feet struggled to carry her heavy body. Her brothers are still active and continue to lose more weight. The whole family is engaged in this healthy life-style since Liana's parents have totally changed their perspective about fitness and nutrition, maintaining a healthy mindset for their healthier family.

Tami is no longer using her pedometer. She knows exactly how to stay active, and what it means for her to take even more than 10,000 steps per day.

Aida is breaking new boundaries now, going on to run 4 kms. three times a week. Her husband is joining her, and as a family they are engaged in a healthy and active life-style. Aida knows she is able to dream about "n'importe quoi" and she can realize those dreams. If she did it with running, she can do it with everything she sets her mind upon.

Barak and his wife are working on a larger family. They have recently returned from China where they took some courses in acupuncture and they travelled together. Their communication has improved for the better, and they are thinking about opening a clinic together.

Tamara has recently made "Aliyah", arriving from California to permanently living in Israel. She is happily married, the mother of a beautiful commercially-photographed baby girl, and her days of anorexia are long forgotten. She is still adjusting to life in Israel, but enjoys her family's love and support. Tamara takes the time to plan her future, maybe as a designer.

Belle and Leroy are working on enlarging their family with the help of a surrogate mother and an egg donation. Belle's heart condition won't allow her to carry a child nor to go through an IVF procedure. With the financial help of her father and after having dealt with all the necessary bureaucracy, she and Leroy are awaiting the stork's arrival.

Irene is no longer a victim of Lupus. Illness and diseases are no longer in her vocabulary as she embraces an active and vigorous (sometimes to the extreme) life-style. She is focusing on her physical activities in hope to never feel weak and helpless, she gets much support and love from her husband and her many friends. Irene wrote me this text message after having completed the 80-km. competitive bike riding:

"There were more than three pretty hard tops to climb; I managed to ride them all. I did it! Two medals I received this week. For running (the 10k Nike run) and this Tour (80 km bicycle ride around the Sea of Galilee). They are the living proof that I am no longer sick, that I replaced Lupus with possibilities, endless possibilities and that, oh yes, I can do it".

All those wonderful people wanted the change and they strove to achieve it. And you, what about you?

Think about a stone tossed into a flat pond. The stone falls gently yet rapidly straight down to the bottom, not before it creates ripples all around. Those ripples continue to grow further and further for a distance, under the influence of that tiny innocent stone you tossed. You cannot predict how many circles are formed or how far the water will take them, but you know you are responsible for that natural reaction of the water, and you know those ripples go farther and farther away conveying the news: "A stone was tossed into the pond". When you take responsibility for your life, your body, your soul, you yourself dive into the depths of your being; you are that tiny stone. Then ripples start to form, thanks to you. You cannot predict their course but you know they are there. So don't just sit there and do nothing except for maybe complaining about life or arguing about your limitations. Your health and happiness are up to you now. You are the one who holds the key to open the door to better health, you have the power to change; you know the secret and the formula for your bright now and a brighter future. And when you do that, know you create many circles around you that slowly yet certainly approach others, enlighten their lives, inspire their soul. You get in touch with your inner compass and get to know yourself. Listen to your body and soul and fulfill its needs. Enjoy the benefits of a "personalized way of life", and go ahead now and enjoy your life. The rest will surely follow.

Bibliography

Fitness

Agin B, and Perkins Sh., Healthy Aging for Dummies, Wily publishing Inc. Indiana, 2008.

Alford, J.W and Malcolm A.R, 1970, Sprinting and Relay Racing, London, Amateur Athletic Association.

Amiri-Khorasani, M, Sotoodeh V Oct. 2013, "The acute effects of combined static and dynamic stretch protocols on fitness performances in soccer players.",' The Journal of Sports Medicine Physical Fitness, 53(5):559-65.

Archer Sh., The Walking Deck: 50 Ways to Walk Yourself Healthy, Chronicle Books LLC 2010.

Arnheim, D.D., Prentice, W.E., Principles of athletic training. 9th ed. McGraw Hill, pp 570-574, 1997.

Astrand, P O, 1976, Textbook of work physiology, New York, MacGraw-Hill Book Company.

Aubrey A, sep 2006, "Chi Runners Poised for Softer Landings", in NPR.org.

Aubrey A, Jul 2006, "Now That's a Stretch! (And it won't Heart a bit)", in NPR.org

Ayan C 2007, "Systemic lupus erythematosus and exercise", in Lupus, 16(1):5-9.

Baggett, K, (n.d.), 2008, "Understanding Muscle Fiber Types", in. Bodybuilding.com. 10-17.

Barnes JN and al, Sep. 2012, " Cardiovascular benefits of habitual exercise in systemic lupus erythematosus: a review", in The Physician and Sports Medicine, 40(3):43-8.

Barnes PM, and al., Dec 2008," Complementary and alternative medicine use among adults and children: United States, 2007", in National Health Statistics Reports, 10;(12):1-23.

Bartenieff, Irmgard, and Dori Lewis, 1980, Body Movement; Coping with the Environment. New York: Gordon and Breach.

Beneka, A. G., et al., 2012, "Muscle performance following an acute bout of plyometric training combined with low or high intensity weight exercise'" in Journal of Sport Sciences, 21, 1-9.

Berset F., Sep., 1992, "Percentage of body fat and risk factors of coronary heart disease", in Tidsskrift For Den Norske Laegeforening 20;112(22):2848-51.

Blair SN, Morris JN, April 2009, "Healthy hearts--and the universal benefits of being physically active: physical activity and health", in Annals of Epidemiology, (4):253-6.

Bloch A., June 1997, The influence of warm-up on achievements and levels of lactic acids in the 400 meters run, Natanya, Wingate Institute. (In Hebrew).

Bonov, P, 1991, "Study of the relationship between speed, heart rate and the accumulation of lactic acid in the blood", IAFF, 6:4: 51-54.

Bompa, T., 1994, Theory and Methodology of Training, the key to athletic performance Dubuques, Iowa: Kendall_hunt Publishing Co.

Bompa T., Mauro Di P. and Lorenzo Cornacchia, (Oct 2, 2002), Serious Strength Training - 2nd edition.

Bompa T., 2006, Total training for coaching team sports, Toronto, Sport Books Publisher.

Bompa T., 1993, Power Training for Sport: Plyometrics for Maximum Power Development, New-York, Mosaic Press.

Booth FW and al, 2000, "Waging war on modern chronic diseases: primary prevention through exercise biology," in Journal of Applied Physiology, vol. 88, no. 2, pp. 774–787, 2000

Booth R., 2010, Who Took My Collagen and How Can I get it Back?, in http://www.thevenusweek.com

Bowley MP and al., Aug. 2010, " Age changes in myelinated nerve fibers of the cingulate bundle and corpus callosum in the rhesus monkey", in The Journal of Comparative Neurology, 1;518(15):3046-64.

Buono MJ, Roby JJ, Micale FG, Sallis JF. (1989), "Predicting maximal oxygen uptake in children: modification of the Astrand-Ryhming test", in Pediatric Exercise Science ;1:278-283.

Brant J, "Look great at any age", in Men's Health, 2010 Rodale Inc, MensHealth.com.

Breitbart R, Fyler, D., 2006, "Tetralogy of Fallot", In Nadas' Pediatric Cardiology, 2ed, Ed. Keane, Locke, & Fyler, Philadelphia: Saunders-Elsevier, , p. 559.

Brickman AM and al., Mar.2007, "An in vivo correlate of exercise-induced neurogenesis in the adult dentate gyrus", in Proceedings of the National Academy of Sciences of the USA, 104(13):5638-43

Brunner RL, et al. 2010, "Menopausal symptom experience before and after stopping estrogen therapy in the Women's Health Initiative randomized, placebo-controlled trial", in. Menopause.;17:946-954.

Burfoot A. (Editor), 2004, Runner's World Complete Book of Running: Everything You Need to Run for Fun, Fitness and Competition, Rodale Books (first published 1997).

Bure Candace C., 2011, Reshaping It All: Motivation for Physical and Spiritual Fitness, by B&H Books, (first published December 20th 2010)

Byberg L and al., March 2009, "Total mortality after changes in leisure time physical activity in 50 year old men: 35 year follow-up of population based cohort", in BMJ Clinical research ed. 5;338:b688.

Carolyn S. Kortge, The Spirited Walker: Fitness Walking For Clarity, Balance, and Spiritual Connection, HarperCollins Publishers, New York, 1998.

Carabello, B. A., 2005,. "Modern Management of Mitral Stenosis". Circulation 112 (3): 432–7

Carvalho MR, and al., Dec., 2005, " Effects of supervised cardiovascular training program on exercise tolerance, aerobic capacity, and quality of life in patients with systemic lupus erythematosus", in Arthritis and Rheumatism, 15;53(6):838-44.

Chumillas S., and al, Jan 1998, "Prevention of postoperative pulmonary complications through respiratory rehabilitation: a controlled clinical study", in Archives of Physical Medicine and Rehabilitation, 79(1):5-9.

Cipriani DJ and al., Sep. 2005, " Backward walking at three levels of treadmill inclination: an electromyographic and kinematic analysis", in The Journal of Orthopaedic and Sports Physical Therapy, 22(3):95-102

Chaput JP and al, 2011, "Physical Activity Plays an Important Role in Body Weight Regulation", in Journal of Obesity, 11 pages.

Chu, D., 1998, "Jumping into plyometrics" (2nd ed. ed.). Champaign, IL: Human Kinetics. pp. 1–4.

Dai T. H., and al., 2001, Relationship between muscle output and functional MRI-measured brain activation. Exp. Brain Res. 140, 290–300.

Davis SR, and al., Nov 2008, "Testosterone for low libido in postmenopausal women not taking estrogen", in New England Journal of Medicine, 6;359(19):2005-17.

Deforche B and al, Sep. 2012, " How to make overweight children exercise and follow the recommendations", in International Journal of Pediatric Obesity, 1:35-41. doi: 10.3109/17477166.2011.583660.

Dreyer D., Chi-Running, A Revolutionary Approach to Effortless Injury-Free Running, ChiLiving, Inc, Asheville, 2009.

Feldman A., (36 articles monthly published from 2009-2012), "Twenty minutes and go'" in Menta Health Magazine, Tel Aviv, Yediot Ahronot. (In Hebrew).

Feldman A., March 2009, "how to change a bad habit using your Mind", in Menta Health Magazine, Tel Aviv, Yediot Ahronot. (In Hebrew)

Fenton M., The complete guide to walking for health, weight loss, and fitness, Guilford CT: Lyon Press, 2001.

Fenton M., Pedometer Walking: Stepping Your Way to Health, Weight Loss, and Fitness, The Lion Press, Connecticut. 2006

Ferrari R, and al, Aud 2013, "Efficiency of twice weekly concurrent training in trained elderly men", in Experimental Gerontology, doi:pii: S0531-5565(13)00237-4. 10.1016/j.exger.2013.07.016

Forte S and al., Dec 1999, "Pulmonary gas exchange and exercise capacity in patients with systemic lupus erythematosus" in The Journal of Rheumatology, 26(12):2591-4.

Fox, L.E, 1984, Sport Physiology 2nd ed. New York Saunders College Publishing.

Frontera WR, 2000, "Aging of skeletal muscle: a 12-yr longitudinal study", in Journal of Applied Physiology ;88:1321–1326

Galloway J, Walking: The Complete Book, Oxford, Meyer & Meyer Sport, (UK), 2006.

Gibala MJ and al, Apr. 2008 "Metabolic adaptations to short-term high-intensity interval training: a little pain for a lot of gain?" in Exercise and sport sciences reviews, ;36(2):58-63. doi: 10.1097/JES.0b013e318168ec1f.

Go AS., and al, Aug., 2007, "Comparative effectiveness of beta-adrenergic antagonists (atenolol, metoprolol tartrate, carvedilol) on the risk of rehospitalization in adults with heart failure", in The American Journal of Cardiology, 100(4):690-6.

Goldenring J, nov. 2011, "Hypotonia", in MedlinePlus the National Institutes of Health's Web , National Library of Medicine San Diego, CA.

Goldfarb HA and Jamurtas AZ., Jul. 1997, "Beta-endorphin response to exercise. An update", in Sports Medicine, 24(1):8-16.

Goran ML, Apr. 1999, " Role of physical activity in the prevention of obesity in children", in International Journal of Obesity and related Metabolic disorders, 23 Suppl 3:S18-33 .

Green JS, Jan. 2002, " Menopause, estrogen, and training effects on exercise hemodynamics: the HERITAGE study", in Medicine and Science in Sports and exercise ;34(1):74-82. .

Guy MS, Sandhu SK, Gowdy JM, Cartier CC, Adams JH. MRI of the axillary arch muscle: prevalence, anatomic relations, and potential consequences. AJR Am J Roentgenol. 2011 Jan;196(1):W52-7.

Harman, E.A.et al., 1991, "Estimation of Human Power Output From Vertical Jump", in .

Journal of Applied Sport Science Research, 5(3), p. 116-120.

Hall JC., and al, Jan. 1996 "Prevention of respiratory complications after abdominal surgery: a randomised clinical trial" in BMJ, 312(7024):148-52; discussion 152-3.

Haruki Murrakami, What I Talk about when I Talk about Running", Keter, Jerusalem, 2005.

Hathaway H, Understanding Your Body Alignment, New Age books, New Delhi, 2000.

Helgerud J, and al, Apr 2007, "Aerobic high-intensity intervals improve VO2max more than moderate training", in Medicine and Science in Sports and Exercise, 39(4):665-71.

Herbert RD and al., Jul. 2011, " Stretching to prevent or reduce muscle soreness after exercise", in Cochrane Database of Systematic Reviews, 6;(7):CD004577

Herring MP., and al., Feb. 2010, "The effect of exercise training on anxiety symptoms among patients: a systematic review", in Archives of Internal Medicine, 22;170(4):321-31

Hodgson J., Mastering Movement: The Life and Work of Rudolf Laban, Routledge, NY, 2001.

Huberty J and al, 2013, "Developing an Instrument to Measure Physical Activity Self-Worth Inventory (WPASWI)", in Psychology of Sport and Exercise, 14(1). DOI:

Hutchinson A., 2011, Which Comes First, Cardio or Weights?: Fitness Myths, Training Truths, and Other Surprising Discoveries from the Science of Exercise, William Morrow Paperbacks.

Ho M and al, Aug. 2013, "Impact of Dietary and Exercise Interventions on Weight Change and Metabolic Outcomes in Obese Children and Adolescents: A Systematic Review and Meta-analysis of Randomized Trials", in JAMA Pediatrics, 1;167(8):759-68. doi: 10.1001/jamapediatrics.2013.1453.

Iscoe. J., (1998). Control of abdominal muscles. Journal of Progress in Neurobiology.(56) 4

Kalman DA, and al., May 1990, " The role of muscle loss in the age-related decline of grip strength: cross-sectional and longitudinal perspectives", in Journal of Gerontology, 45(3):M82-8.

Kent Rush A., The way of stretching, flexibility for body and mind" Hachette, NY, 2005.

Kats L. D, 2002 The Way to Eat: A Six-Step Path to Lifelong Weight Control, Illinois, Sourcebooks.

Kavalso A., (2011), "Natural movement and Functional Exercise", in http://www.alkavadlo.com/2011/09/16/natural-movement-and-functional-exercise/

Kirk I E and al, March 2013, " Physical activity and brain plasticity in late adulthood", in

Dialogues in Clinical Neuroscience, 15(1): 99–108.

Kraemer WJ and al, Feb. 1998, "Acute hormonal responses to heavy resistance exercise in younger and older men", in European Journal of Applied Physiology and Occupational Physiology, 77(3):206-11.

Kwok TC., and al., 2011, " Effectiveness of coordination exercise in improving cognitive function in older adults: a prospective study", in Clinical interventions in Aging, 10.2147/CIA.S19883

Lawrence H. Kushi ScD and al, (Jan 2012), "American Cancer Society guidelines on nutrition and physical activity for cancer prevention; Reducing the risk of cancer with healthy food choices and physical activity" in CA, The Cancer Journal for Clinicians, DOI: 10.3322/caac.20140

Lebon F and al., Apr. 2008, "Modulation of EMG power spectrum frequency during motor imagery", in Neuroscience letters, 435(3):181-5 .

Lebon F and al., Jun. 2010, "Benefits of motor imagery training on muscle strength", in Journal of Strength and Conditioning Research, 24(6):1680-7.

Lee Goss D, A Comparison of Lower Extremity Join Work and Initial Loading Rates among Four different Running Style, UMI, 2012.

Legge and Banister, The Astrand-Ryhming nomogram revisited J Appl Physiol.1986; 61: 1203-1209.

Lindsay Bruce, MD, "Premature Ventricular Contractions", HealthHub from Cleverland Clinic, 2013.

Source: http://my.clevelandclinic.org/heart/disorders/electric/premature-ventricular-contractions.aspx

Little John R. and Sharkey, J. The Wisdom Of Mike Mentzer The Art, Science, And Philosophy Of A Bodybuilding Legend, McGraw-Hill Companies, 2007.

Liu-Ambrose T., and al., Jan. 2010, " Resistance training and executive functions: a 12-month randomized controlled trial", in Archives of Internal Medicine 25;170(2):170-8.

Manini TM and al, Oct. 2012, " Growth hormone responses to acute resistance exercise with vascular restriction in young and old men", in Growth Hormone and IGF Research .;22(5):167-72. doi: 10.1016/j.ghir.2012.05.002

LeMura LM and al, Sep. 2011, "Treadmill and cycle ergometry testing in 5- to 6-year-old children", in European Journal of applied physiology, 85(5):472-8.

Malouin F., and Richards C, Fab. 2010, "Mental Practice for Relearning Locomotor Skills", in Physical Therapy Journal, 90: (2) 240-251.

Marcus et al, (2008), "Comparison of Combined Aerobic and High-Force Eccentric Resistance Exercise With Aerobic Exercise Only for People With Type 2 Diabetes Mellitus", in Physical Therapy; DOI: 10.2522/ptj.20080124

Masalgin N.A. and al, 1987, "The Influence of the Shock Method of Training on the Electromyographic Parameters of Explosive Effort". Teoriya i Praktika Fizicheskoi Kultury (Theory and Practice of Physical Culture) 1. pp. 45–46.

Mathers DC., and al., 2002, "Global patterns of healthy life expectancy for older women", in Journal of Women and Aging, 14(1-2):99-117.

McPhee JS., and al,Jun 2013, "Physiological and functional evaluation of healthy young and older men and women: design of the European MyoAge study",in Biogerontology, 14(3):325-37. doi: 10.1007/s10522-013-9434-7

McGinnis JM, Foege WH., 1993, "Actual causes of death in the United States" in JAMA.; 270: 2207-2212.

Mc Quaide-Little K, 2012, "Anti-Aging Effects of Exercise", in Sports Science Institute of South Africa, http://www.ssisa.com/articles/exercise/anti-ageing-effects-of-exercise---by-kathleen-mc-quaide-little/

Meyers C., Walking, a complete guide to a complete exercise, Ballantine Books, New York, 2007

Michaels J., 2007, Making the Cut: The 30-Day Diet and Fitness Plan for the Strongest, Sexiest You, Harmony.

Moore, Carol Lynne, 1982, Executives in Action: A Guide to Balanced Decision–making in Management. Estover, Plymouth: MacDonald & Evans. (First published as Action Profiling, 1978.)

Moore, Carol Lynne and Kaoru Yamamoto, 1988, Beyond Words. New York: Gordon and Breach.

Moore PM, Dec. 1998, "A workplace stretching program. Physiologic and perception measurements before and after participation", in Official Journal of the American Association of Occupational Health Nurses, 46(12):563-8.

Morgan Al and al, May 2010, "Walking toward a new me: the impact of prescribed walking 10,000 steps/day on physical and psychological well-being", in Journal of Physical Activity and health, 7(3):299-307.

Nelson HD., Mar. 2008, "Menopause", in Lancet, 1;371(9614):760-70.

Nilsson N, Mad Scientist Muscle: Build "Monster" Mass with Science-Based Training, Priced World Publishing, Chicago, 2012.

Nguyen MN., and al, Aug. 1997, "Regular exercise in 30- to 60-year-old men: combining the stages-of-change model and the theory of planned behavior to identify determinants for targeting heart health interventions", in Journal of Community Health, 22(4):233-46

Nummela, T., Vuorinaa and Rusko, H, 1991, "Changes in force production, blood lactate and EMG activity in the 400 m sprint" in Journal of sport science, 10, 217-228.

O'Donnell DE, McGuire M, Samis L, Webb KA. General exercise training improves ventilatory and peripheral muscle strength and endurance in chronic airflow limitation. Am J Respir Crit Care Med. 1998;157:1489–97

Oliverdia R., and al., Dec. 2005, "Clinical features of muscle dysmorphia among males with body dysmorphic disorder", in Body Image ;2(4):395-400.

Oriel KN and al, 2011, " The effects of aerobic exercise on academic engagement in young children with autism spectrum disorder", in, Pediatric Physical Therapy, 23(2):187-93. doi: 10.1097/PEP.0b013e318218f149.

Paoli A., and al, 2012, " High-Intensity Interval Resistance Training (HIRT) influences resting energy expenditure and respiratory ratio in non-dieting individuals", in Journal of Translational Medicine, doi:10.1186/1479-5876-10-237.

Paton, C and al., 2004, "Effects of High-intensity Training on Performance and Physiology of Endurance Athletes." In Sportscience 8, 25-40.

Perrig-Chiello P., and al., Jul 1998, " The effects of resistance training on well-being and memory in elderly volunteers", in Age and Aging, 27(4):469-75.

Perry CG, and al, Dec. 2008, "High-intensity aerobic interval training increases fat and carbohydrate metabolic capacities in human skeletal muscle", in Applied Physiology Nutrition and Metabolism, 33(6):1112-23. doi: 10.1139/H08-097.

Phelan S and l, Apr. 2006, " Are the eating and exercise habits of successful weight losers changing?" in Obesity, 14(4):710-6.

Pines A., Berry EM Oct., 2007' " Exercise in the menopause - an update", in Climacteric: the Journal of the International Menopause society, 2:42-6.

Pontifex MB and al, Mar 2013, "Exercise improves behavioral, neurocognitive, and scholastic performance in children with attention-deficit/hyperactivity disorder", in Journal of Pediatrics 162(3):543-51. doi: 10.1016/j.jpeds.2012.08.036. Epub 2012 Oct 17.

Poole, RM, ed., 1986, The Incredible Machine. Washington, DC: National Geographic Society. pp. 307–311.

Praag, H. van, 2009, "Exercise and the brain: something to chew on," Trends in Neurosciences, vol. 32, no. 5, pp. 283–290.

Rafael F and Al, (April 2010), "Core Muscle Activation During Swiss Ball and Traditional Abdominal Exercises", Journal of Orthpaedic & Sport Physical Therapy ;40(5):265-276.

Raley J, Spark: The Revolutionary New Science of Exercise and the Brain, Little Brown and Company, NY, 2008.

Randlov A., et al. , Intensive dynamic training for females with chronic neck/shoulder pain. A randomized controlled trial. Clin Rehabil, 1998. 12(3): p. 200–10.

Ranganathan V. K., Siemionow V., Liu J. Z., Sahgal V., Yue G. H., (2004), "From mental power to muscle power – gaining strength by using the mind", Neuropsychologia 42, 944–956

Ramsey-Goldman R. and al., Oct. 2000, "A pilot study on the effects of exercise in patients with systemic lupus erythematosus", In Arthritis Care and Research 13(5):262-9.

Ranganathan VK and al., 2004, "From mental power to muscle power--gaining strength by using the mind" in Neuropsychologia, 42(7):944-56.

Ravussin, E and Elliot Danforth Jr.*, jan 1999, "Beyond Sloth--Physical Activity and Weight Gain", in HUMAN PHYSIOLOGY Vol. 283 no. 5399 pp. 184-185.

Ravussin, E, 2005, "A NEAT Way to Control Weight?"" in Science 28 Vol. 307 no. 5709 pp. 530-531

Raz N and Lindenberger U., March 2010, "The news of cognitive cure for age-related brain shrinkage is premature. A comment on Burgmans et al", in Neuropsychology, 24 (2): 255-257.

RE Cink and TR Thomas, 1981, "Validity of the Astrand-Ryhming nomogram for predicting maximal oxygen intake", in British Journal of Sports Medicine, Vol 15, Issue 3 182-185.

Reily, T Secher, N, Snell, P& Williams, L, 1990, Physiology of sports, London e & F.N Spon.

Reiser ., and al., (2011) "Strength Gains by Motor Imagery with Different Ratios of Physical to Mental Practice", in Frontiers in Psychology, 2: 194.

Ries N M and Tigerstrom B V, April 2010, "Roadblocks to laws for healthy eating and activity", in Canadian Medical Association, 182:687-692; published ahead of print February 16, 2010, doi:10.1503/cmaj.091403

Ruiz IrastorzaG., and al., Jan. 2010, "Clinical efficacy and side effects of antimalarials in systemic lupus erythematosus: a systematic review", in Annuals of the Rheumatic Diseases. 69(1):20-8. doi: 10.1136/ard.2008.101766.

Robin M Daly and al., 2013, " Gender specific age-related changes in bone density, muscle strength and functional performance in the elderly: a-10 year prospective population-based study", in BMC Geriatrics 13:71 doi:10.1186/1471-2318-13-71

Rogers MA, Evans WJ., 1993, "Changes in skeletal muscle with aging: effects of exercise training", in Exercise Sports and Science; 21:65–102

Rotstein A, 1994, Biology and Physiology of Exercise, Natanya, Wingate Ins. (In Hebrew)

Runnels ED., and al, 2005 " Influence of age on isometric, isotonic, and isokinetic force production characteristics in men", in Journal of Geriatric Physical therapy, 28(3):74-84.

Sahai A, 2007, " Dentate gyrus neurogenesis and depression", in Progress in Brain Research, 163:697-722.

Shabir Bhimji, 2013, "Tetralogy of Fallot", in Medscape Reference, http://emedicine.medscape.com/article/2035949-overview.

Shahidi B, Haight A, Maluf K., (jun 22, 2013), "Differential effects of mental concentration and acute psychosocial stress on cervical muscle activity and posture", in Journal of Electromyography and Kinesiology, PII: S1050-6411(13)00123-5.

Shepard JC, 1994, Aerobic Fitness and health, Champaign, IL Human Kinetics Publishers Inc.

Sidman C, Corbin CB, LeMasurier G, "promoting physical activity among sedentary women using pedometers" in Research Quarterly for exercise and Sport, 75: 122-129, 2004.

Sidman C. "Count your steps to health and fitness" in American College of Sports and Medicine's Health and Fitness Journal 6 (I): 13-17, 2002.

Siler B., the Pilates Body, the ultimate at home guide to strengthening and toning your body without machines, Broadway Books, 2000.

Sivakumar G, and al, Apr. 2011, "Acute effects of deep breathing for a short duration (2-10 minutes) on pulmonary functions in healthy young volunteers", in Indian Journal of Physiology and Pharmacology, 55(2):154-9.

Sinha-Hikim I., and al., Jul. 2002, "Testosterone-induced increase in muscle size in healthy young men is associated with muscle fiber hypertrophy", in American Journal of Physiology ;283(1):E154-64.

Sinha S., and al,Dec., 2007, " Improvement of glutathione and total antioxidant status with yoga", in Journal of Alternative and Complementary medicine 13(10):1085-90 .

Small K., and al. 2008," A systematic review into the efficacy of static stretching as part of a warm-up for the prevention of exercise-related injury", in Research in Sports Medicine, 16(3):213-31

Streeter CC., and al., Nov. 2010, " Effects of yoga versus walking on mood, anxiety, and brain GABA levels: a randomized controlled MRS study" in Journal of Alternative and Complementary medicine, 16(11):1145-52

Strombeck B and al., March 2007, " The role of exercise in the rehabilitation of patients with systemic lupus erythematosus and patients with primary Sjögren's syndrome", in Current Opinion on Rheumatology, 19(2):197-203.

Strong WB, and al, Jun 2005, " Evidence based physical activity for school-age youth", in The Journal of Pediatrics, 146(6):732-7.

Thomas JA, McIntosh JM., Jan. 1994, "Are incentive spirometry, intermittent positive pressure breathing, and deep breathing exercises effective in the prevention of postoperative pulmonary complications after upper abdominal surgery? A systematic overview and meta-analysis including commentary by Dean E with author response", in Physical Therapy, 74(1):3–16.

Toth MJ., and al., 2006 "Role of ovarian hormones in the regulation of protein metabolism in women: effects of menopausal status and hormone replacement therapy" in American Journal of Physiology, 291: E639-E646.

Toth MJ., and al., Aug. 1999, "Hormonal and Physiological Correlates of Energy Expenditure and Substrate Oxidation in Middle-Aged, Premenopausal Women", in The Journal of Clinical Endocrinology & Metabolism 84 no. 8 2771-2775.

Talanian JL, Apr. 2007, "Two weeks of high-intensity aerobic interval training increases the capacity for fat oxidation during exercise in women", in Journal of Applied Physiology, 102(4):1439-47

Teegarden D., May 1995, "Peak bone mass in young women", in Journal of Bone and Mineral Research, 10(5):711-5.

Tench CM and al., Sep. 2003, " Fatigue in systemic lupus erythematosus: a randomized controlled trial of exercise", in Rheumatology (Oxford, England), 42(9):1050-4. Epub 2003 Apr 16.

Thornton EV and al., 2004 " Health benefits of Tai Chi exercise: improved balance and blood pressure in middle-aged women", in Health Promotion International, 19 (1): 33-38.

Tofthagen C., Sep. 2012, " Strength and balance training for adults with peripheral neuropathy and high risk of fall: current evidence and implications for future research", in Oncology Nursing Forum, 39(5):E416-24.

Tussing-Humphreys Land al, (Jun 6 2013), "A church-based diet and physical activity intervention for rural, lower Mississippi Delta African American adults: delta body and soul effectiveness study, 2010-2011", in Prevention Chronic Disease, 10:E92. doi: 10.5888/pcd10.120286.

Uramoto AM, Jan. 1999, "Trends in the incidence and mortality of systemic lupus erythematosus, 1950-1992", in Arthritis and Rheumatism, 42(1):46-50.

Vindum T., Outdoor Fitness, Falcon Guides, Montana, 2009.

Watts Emily,2009, I Hate It When Exercise Is the Answer: A Fitness Program for the Soul, Deseret Book.

Westerdahl E, and al., Nov. 2005, "Deep-breathing exercises reduce atelectasis and improve pulmonary function after coronary artery bypass surgery", in Chest 128:3482–8.

Tudor Lock C. "Taking steps towards increased physical activity: using pedometers to measure and motivate", in Research Digest 3 (17). June 2002.

Tudor-Locke Catrine, Manpo-Kei, The Art and Science of Steps Counting. Victoria, BC; Trafford Publishing, 2003.

Ullmann, Lisa (1975). Some hints for the student of movement. In Modern Educational Dance, by R. Laban; 3rd edition revised and edited by L. Ullmann (pp. 108-134). London: MacDonald & Evans.

Verkhoshansky Y and , Verkhoshansky N (2011). Specialized Strength and Conditioning, Manual For Coaches. Verkhoshansky SSTM

Vinoth K. and al., 2004), "From mental power to muscle power; gaining strength by using the mind", in Neuropsychologia ,42, 944-150;956

Vispute SS and al, Sep 2011, " The effect of abdominal exercise on abdominal fat", in Journal of Strength and Conditioning Research, (9):2559-64.

Science Daily: Exercise Important In Reducing Size Of Abdominal Fat Cells. Preliminary reports on a study, 7 August 2006.

Singh VP and al., Jul-Sep 2011, "Effects of upper body resistance training on pulmonary functions in sedentary male smokers", in International Journal of Sports Physical Therapy, (3): 169-173.

Waenher P., March 2010, "Pyramid Training", about.com guide.

Watts K and al, 2005, " Exercise training in obese children and adolescents: current concepts, in Sports Medicine, 35(5):375-92.

Wells, K.F. & Dillon, E.K. 1952, "The sit and reach. A test of back and leg flexibility", in . Research Quarterly, 23. 115-118.

Wezenberg D and al, apr 2011, "Mind your step: metabolic energy cost while walking an enforced gait pattern", in Gait Posture, 33(4):544-9.

Wikgren J. and al, (may 2012) " Selective breeding for endurance running capacity affects cognitive but not motor learning in rats.", in Physiology and Behavior, vol 106 (2), 95-100.

Wiley J & Sons, Ltd (Published by), Nov. 2011, "Exercise for improving balance in older people, in Cochrane Database of Systematic Reviews: Plain Language Summaries.

Winter DA and al,, Spt. 1989 "Backward walking: a simple reversal of forward walking?", in Journal of Motor behavior, 21(3):291-305.

Woods K., and al., 2007, "Warm-up and stretching in the prevention of muscular injury", in Sports Medicine, 37(12):1089-99.

Yang YR., and al, May 2005 " Gait outcomes after additional backward walking training in patients with stroke: a randomized controlled trial", in Clinical Rehabilitation, 19(3):264-73.

Ylinen J., et al. , Active neck muscle training in the treatment of chronic neck pain in women: a randomized controlled trial. JAMA, 2003. 289(19): p. 2509–16.

Yeager S, 2011, "Power Walking", in Prevention, www.prevention.com.

Yue G and Cole KJ., May 1992, " Strength increases from the motor program: comparison of training with maximal voluntary and imagined muscle contractions", in Journal of Neurophysiology 67(5):1114-23.

Zeno SA, and al., Jul 2013, "Warm-ups for military fitness testing: rapid evidence assessment of the literature.", in Medicine and Science in Sports and Exercise, 45(7):1369-76.

Mayo clinic staff, Slide show: Exercises to improve your core strength, august 2011. http://www.mayoclinic.com/health/core-strength/SM00047.

Cedric X. Bryant, PhD, chief exercise physiologist, American Council on Exercise, San Diego. Tworoger, S. Sleep, 2003; vol 27, pp. 830-836.

WebMD Medical News: "6 Secrets of Successful Weight Loss."

MyPyramid.gov: "How many calories does physical activity use?" WebMD Medical News: "Yoga May Prevent Weight Gain in Middle Age."Reviewed on August 31, 2010.

Nutrition

Ajja R and al, (Sept. 2012) "Healthy Afterschool Activity and Nutrition Documentation (HAAND)", in Active Living Research, http://activelivingresearch.org/

Airola P., Worldwide Secrets for Staying Young, Health Plus Pub, 1982.

Agus D.B, The End Of Illness, Simon & Schuster Inc., New York, 2012.

Alpert SS., Mar 2005, "A limit on the energy transfer rate from the human fat store in hypophagia", in Journal of Theoretical Biology, 7;233(1):1-13.

Argo CM, and al, Nov 2012, "Weight loss resistance: a further consideration for the nutritional management of obese Equidae", in Veterinary Journal, 194(2):179-88.

Astorino TA, and Roberson DW., Jan 2010, "Efficacy of acute caffeine ingestion for short-term high-intensity exercise performance: a systematic review", in Journal of Strength and Conditioning research, 24(1):257-65..

Attia E ,2010, "Anorexia Nervosa: Current Status and Future Directions", in Annual Review of Medicine 61 (1): 425–35.

Augustin LS, and al, Apr. 2004, "Glycemic index, glycemic load and risk of gastric cancer", in Annals of Oncology, Official Journal of the European Society for Medical Oncology, 15(4):581-4.

Augustus-Horvath CL, Tylka TL., Jan 2011, "The acceptance model of intuitive eating: a comparison of women in emerging adulthood, early adulthood, and middle adulthood", in Journal of Counseling Psychology, 58(1):110-25.

Avalos L, Tylka TL, Wood-Barcalow N.Sep 2005, "The Body Appreciation Scale: development and psychometric evaluation", in Body Image, 2(3):285-97.

Balch Phyllis A., 2006, Prescription for Nutritional Healing: A Practical A-to-Z Reference to Drug-Free Remedies Using Vitamins, Minerals, Herbs & Food Supplements, Avery Trade. (First published January 1st 1991).

Barlow SE Expert Committee, Dec 2007, "Expert committee recommendations regarding the prevention, assessment, and treatment of child and adolescent overweight and obesity: summary report" in Pediatrics, 120 Suppl 4:S164-92.

Benelam B., May 2009, "Satiation, satiety and their effects on eating behavior", in Nutrition Bulletin, 34, 126–173.

Benton D, and al, Nov 2007, "The influence of the glycemic load of breakfast on the behavior of children in school", in Physiology and Behavior, 23;92(4):717-24 .

Berenson GS, and al, Oct 1992, "Atherosclerosis of the aorta and coronary arteries and cardiovascular risk factors in persons aged 6 to 30 years and studied at necropsy (The Bogalusa Heart Study)", in The American Journal of Cardiology, 1;70(9):851-8.

Berenson GS and al, Nov 2001, "Bogalusa Heart Study: a long-term community study of a rural biracial (Black/White) population", in The American Journal of the Medical Sciences, 322(5):293-300.

Bergeron D, and Tylka TL. Sep 2007, "Support for the uniqueness of body dissatisfaction from drive for muscularity among men", in Body Image, 4(3):288-95.

Beridot-Therond ME,, Arts I, Fantino M, De La Gueronniere V., Aug 1998, "Short-term effects of the flavour of drinks on ingestive behaviours in man", in Appetite, 31(1):67-81.

Bixler EO, and al., Qug. 2005, " Excessive daytime sleepiness in a general population sample: the role of sleep apnea, age, obesity, diabetes, and depression" in The Journal of Clinical Endocrinology and Metabolism, 90(8):4510-5.

Bonci L, Active Calorie Diet, Rodale Books, PA, 2011.

Bostick RM and al, Jan 1994, "Sugar, meat, and fat intake, and non-dietary risk factors for colon cancer incidence in Iowa women (United States)", in Cancer Causes and Control.;5(1):38-52.

Bower B., and al, Jun 2010, "Poor reported sleep quality predicts low positive affect in daily life among healthy and mood-disordered persons", in Journal of Sleep Research, 19(2):323-32.

Brand-Miller J. and al , The Low GL diet Revolution, the definitive Science-based Weigh Loss Plan, New-York, Marlowe and Company 2005.

Brown R and Ogden J, 2004, "Children's eating attitudes and behaviour: a study of the modelling and control theories of parental influence", in Health Education Research, 19 (3): 261-271.

Burke LM., Dec 2008, "Caffeine and sports performance", in Applies Physiology, Nutrition and Metabolism, 33(6):1319-34.

Butte NF and al., march 2003, "Energy requirements of women of reproductive age", in American Journal of clinical Nutrition vol. 77 no. 3 630-638.

Carnethon MR, and al, Aug. 2012, "Association of weight status with mortality in adults with incident diabetes", in JAMA, the journal of the American Medical Association, 8;308(6):581-90.

Casazza K. and al, (Jan 2013), "Myths, Presumptions, and Facts about Obesity", in The New England Journal of Medicine, ; 368:446-454, DOI: 10.1056/NEJMsa1208051

Chaput JP, and al, 2007, "Psychobiological effects observed in obese men experiencing body weight loss plateau", in Depression and Anxiety, 24(7):518-21.

Chaput JP and al.(2011), "Physical Activity Plays an Important Role in Body Weight Regulation", in Journal of Obesity, Article ID, 11 pages.

Chavarro JE, and al, Nov 2007, "Diet and lifestyle in the prevention of ovulatory disorder infertility", in Obstetrics and Gynecology, 110(5):1050-8.

Chen J and al., Aug. 1998, "A prospective study of N-acetyltransferase genotype, red meat intake, and risk of colorectal cancer", In *Cancer Research* 1;58(15):3307-11.

Chernoff R., Dec 2004, "Protein and older adults", in Journal of the American College of Nutrition, 23(6 Suppl).

Choi KM, and al., Sep. 2013," Higher mortality in metabolically obese normal-weight people than in metabolically healthy obese subjects in elderly Koreans", in Clinical Endocrinology, 79(3):364-70.

Clark N., 2003 , Nancy Clark's Sports Nutrition Guidebook, Human Kinetics Publishers.

Clarkson TB, and al (Collaborators : 37), Jul 2011, "The role of soy isoflavones in menopausal health: report of The North American Menopause Society/Wulf H. Utian Translational Science Symposium in Chicago, IL (October 2010)", in Menopause.;18(7):732-53.

Cleator J and al, Sep. 2012, "Night eating syndrome: implications for severe obesity", in Nutrition and Diabetes, 2(9): e44. doi: 10.1038/nutd.2012.16.

Cohen D., and Farley TA., Jan 2008, "Eating as an automatic behavior", in Preventing Chronic Disease, 5(1):A23.C

Cohen DA,, and Babey SH., Sep 2012, "Contextual influences on eating behaviours: heuristic processing and dietary choices", in Obesity Reviews, an official Journal of the International Association for the Study of Obesity, 13(9):766-79. .

Collins N., Sep 2012, "Why dieting is all in the timing", in The Telegraph, http://www.telegraph.co.uk.

Connor JR, and Menzies SL.Jun 1996, "Relationship of iron to oligodendrocytes and myelination", in Gila, 17(2):83-93.

Conus F., and al, Feb. 2007, "Characteristics of metabolically obese normal-weight (MONW) subjects", in *Applied Physiology, Nutrition and Metabolism*, 32 (1):4-12.

Coronado GD, Beasley J, Livaudais J., Sep-Oct 2011, "Alcohol consumption and the risk of breast cancer", in Salud Publica de Mexico, ;53(5):440-7.

Davison K, Birch L. (2001), "Weight status, parent reaction and self-concept in five-year-old girls", Pediatrics ;107:46–53.

Davison KK, and Birch LL, Aug 2001, "Childhood overweight: a contextual model and recommendations for future research", in Obesity reviews, 2(3):159-71.

Dexter C. and al, April 2013, "Body mass index and incident coronary heart disease in women: a population-based prospective study", in BMC Medicine, 11:87 doi:10.1186/1741-7015-11-87.

Douglas CC., and al, Apr 2007, "Ability of the Harris Benedict formula to predict energy requirements differs with weight history and ethnicity", in Nutrition Research, 27(4): 194–199.

Dulloo AG, and al, Dec 1999, "Efficacy of a green tea extract rich in catechin polyphenols and caffeine in increasing 24-h energy expenditure and fat oxidation in humans", in The American Journal of Clinical Nutrition, 70(6):1040-5.

Eckel, R H., May 2008, "Nonsurgical Management of Obesity in Adults", in New England Journal of Medicine, 358:1941-1950.

Eppley KR, and al, Nov. 1989, "Differential effects of relaxation techniques on trait anxiety: a meta-analysis", in Journal of Clinical Psychology, 45(6):957-74.

Essa MM, and al, Sep 2012, "Neuroprotective effect of natural products against Alzheimer's disease", in Neurochemical Research.;37(9):1829-42.

Epstein M., Dalai Lama XIV (Foreword), 1996, Thoughts Without A Thinker: Psychotherapy From A Buddhist Perspective, Basic Books.

Etminan M, Takkouche B, Caamaño-Isorna F., Mar 2004, "The role of tomato products and lycopene in the prevention of prostate cancer: a meta-analysis of observational studies", in Cancer Epidemiology, biomarkers and prevention, 13(3):340-5.

Fernandez ML Jan 2006, "Dietary cholesterol provided by eggs and plasma lipoproteins in healthy populations", in Current Opinion in Clinical Nutrition and Metabolic care, 9(1):8-12..

Ferraro KF, Thorpe RJ Jr, Wilkinson JA. (2003), "The life course of severe obesity: does childhood overweight matter?" in Journal of Gerontology: Social Sciences 2003;58B(2):S110–S119.

Flegal K. M and al, (Jan 2013), "Association of All-Cause Mortality With Overweight and Obesity Using Standard Body Mass Index Categories : A Systematic Review and Meta-analysis", in JAMA,.;309(1):71-82. doi:10.1001/jama.2012.113905.

Foster-Powell K and al, July 2002, "International table of glycemic index and glycemic load values: 2002", in The American Journal of Clinical Nutrition, 76(1):5-56.

Frankenfield DC., and al., Apr 1998, "The Harris-Benedict studies of human basal metabolism: history and limitations", in Journal of the American Dietetic Association, 98(4):439-45.

Freedman DS, and al, 1999, "The relation of overweight to cardiovascular risk factors among children and adolescents: The Bogalusa Heart Study", in Pediatrics; 103: 1175–1182.

Frechman R, The Food is My Friend Diet, Gales Publishing, Burbank, California, 2012.

Froy O., Sep. 2013, "Circadian aspects of energy metabolism and aging", in Ageing Research Reviews, S1568-1637(13)00065-2.

Fung T., and al, Feb. 2003, "Major dietary patterns and the risk of colorectal cancer in women", in Achieves of Internal Medicine, 10;163(3):309-14.

Gallop Rick, 2004, Living the Glycemic Index Diet, Delicious Recipes and Real-Life Strategies to lose weight and keep it off, New-York, Workman Publishing.

Gangwisch JE, and al, Oct 2005, " Inadequate sleep as a risk factor for obesity: analyses of the NHANES I.", in Sleep, 28(10):1289-96.

Garaulet M, and al, Feb 2011, "Ghrelin, sleep reduction and evening preference: relationships to CLOCK 3111 T/C SNP and weight loss", in PLoS One, 28;6(2):e17435. doi: 10.1371/journal.pone.0017435.

Gardener H, and al, Sep 2012, "Diet soft drink consumption is associated with an increased risk of vascular events in the Northern Manhattan Study", in Journal of General Internal Medicine, 27(9):1120-6.

German JB, and Walzem RL., 2000, "The health benefits of wine", in Annual Review of Nutrition, 20:561-93.

Gibson EL, Wardle J, Watts CJ., Oct 1998, "Fruit and vegetable consumption, nutritional knowledge and beliefs in mothers and children",, in Appetite, 31(2):205-28.

Glade MJ., Oct 2010, "Caffeine-Not just a stimulant", in Nutrition, 26(10):932-8.

Glanz K, and al, Aug. 1997, "Are awareness of dietary fat intake and actual fat consumption associated?--a Dutch-American comparison", in European Journal of Clinical Nutrition, 51(8):542-7.

Golan M and Crow S. Feb 2004, "Targeting parents exclusively in the treatment of childhood obesity: long-term results", in Obesity Research, 12(2):357-61.

Goncalves MD, and al., May 2009, "The treatment of night eating: the patient's perspective", in European Eating Disorders Review, The Journal of the Eating Disorders Association, 17(3):184-90. doi: 10.1002/erv.918.

Graham TE., 2001, "Caffeine and exercise: metabolism, endurance and performance", in Sports Medicine, 31(11):785-807.

Graham DJ and Laska MN, Mar 2012, "Nutrition label use partially mediates the relationship between attitude toward healthy eating and overall dietary quality among college students", in Journal of the Academy of Nutrition and Dietetics, 112(3):414-8.

Greenberg JA,, Boozer CN, Geliebter A., Oct 2006, "Coffee, diabetes, and weight control", in The American Journal of Clinical Nutrition, 84(4):682-93.

Grenville M., Natural Solutions to Menopause, Pan Macmillan, 2013.

Haiken M, Jul 2013, "Weight Loss After 40 -- Why It's So Hard, and What Works", in Caring.com

Hart D, Weight Loss Ladder - 10 steps to lasting weight loss and happiness, TM 2013, Kindle version.

Hensrud .D ed., "The Mayo Clinic Diet", Rosetta Books, NY, 2011.

Hill O J and al, Nov 2009, " Using the Energy Gap to Address Obesity: A Commentary", in Journal of the American Dietetic Association, 109 (11), 1848-1853.

Hill P., Nov-Dec. 1991, "It is not what you eat, but how you eat it digestion, life-style, nutrition", in Nutrition, 7(6):385-95.

Hockenbury, Don and Hockenbury, Sandra, Psychology. Worth Publishers, New York. 2008.

Hodgson AB,, Randell RK,, Jeukendrup AE., 2013, "The metabolic and performance effects of caffeine compared to coffee during endurance exercise", in PLoS One.;8(4):e59561.

Holick MF., Dec 2004, "Sunlight and vitamin D for bone health and prevention of autoimmune diseases, cancers, and cardiovascular disease", in The American Journal of Clinical Nutrition, 80(6 Suppl):1678S-88S.

Huang TT., and al, Nov 2004, "Reading nutrition labels and fat consumption in adolescents", in The Journal of Adolescents Health, 35(5):399-401.

Hyman M., The Blood Sugar Solution, Little, Brown and Company, NY, 2012.

Kaizer L, and al, 1989, "Fish consumption and breast cancer risk: an ecological study", in Nutrition and Cancer, 12(1):61-8.

Katcher H I, and al, Jan. 2008, " The effects of a whole grain–enriched hypocaloric diet on cardiovascular disease risk factors in men and women with metabolic syndrome1", in American Society for Clinical Nutrition, vol. 87 no. 1 79-90.

Katz DL., and al. Nov. 2011, " Cocoa and chocolate in human health and disease" in Antioxidants and Redox Signaling 15(10):2779-811.

Kabat G, June 2013, "How Useful Is Body Mass Index In Predicting Long-Term Health?", post at Forbes.com.

Kaizer L., and al., 1989, "Fish consumption and breast cancer risk: an ecological study", in Nutrition and Cancer, 12(1):61-8.

Kannappan R, and al, Oct. 2011, "Neuroprotection by spice-derived nutraceuticals: you are what you eat!", in Molecular Neurobiology, 44(2):142-59.

Kaunitz AM, and al, Aug 2006, Bone mineral density in women aged 25-35 years receiving depot medroxyprogesterone acetate: recovery following discontinuation", in Contraception.;74(2):90-9.

Keen CL., Oct. 2001, " Chocolate: food as medicine/medicine as food" in Journal of the American College of Nutrition, 20(5 Suppl):436S-439S; discussion 440S-442S.

Keizer A, and al, Nov 2011, "Tactile body image disturbance in anorexia nervosa", Psychiatry research, 30;190(1):115-20.

Kornhauser C, and al, Jul-Aug 1994, "[High prevalence of arterial hypertension in women over 50 years of age in the city of Leon, Guanajuato]", [Article in Spanish], in Revista de investigacion Clinica, 46(4):287-94.

Kravits, Len, May 2007, "Winning at Losing: Secrets of Long-Term Weight Loss",in IDEA Fitness Journal, Volume 4, Number 5.

Kreuter MW., and al, Jul-Aug 1997, "Do nutrition label readers eat healthier diets? Behavioral correlates of adults' use of food labels", in American Journal of Preventive Medicine, 13(4):277-83.

Kotz CM, and al, march 2008, "Neuroregulation of nonexercise activity thermogenesis and obesity resistance", in American Journal of Physiology - Regulatory, Integrative and Comparative Vol..294.

Kopelman PG, Grace C, (2004), "New thoughts in managing obesity", Gut, 53: 1044-1053.

Kurzer MS., Oct 2008, "Soy consumption for reduction of menopausal symptoms", in Inflammopharmacology.;16(5):227-9.

Kushi L., H., and al, May 1999, "Prospective Study of Diet and Ovarian Cancer", in American Journal of Epidemiology, V149, Issue 1 Pp. 21-31.

Kwak SM, and al, Korean Meta-analysis Study Group. May 2012, "Efficacy of omega-3 fatty acid supplements (eicosapentaenoic acid and docosahexaenoic acid) in the secondary prevention of cardiovascular disease: a meta-analysis of randomized, double-blind, placebo-controlled trials", in Achieves of Internal Medicine, 14;172(9):686-94.

Hart CN, (October 2011), "Eating and activity habits of overweight children on weekdays and weekends", Int J Pediatr Obes. 6(5-6):467-72.

In-iw S, Manaboriboon B, Chomchai C., Apr 2010, "A comparison of body-image perception, health outlook and eating behavior in mildly obese versus moderately-to-severely obese adolescents", in Journal of the Medical Association of Thailand, 93(4):429-35.

Kenny LC, and al, 2013, "Advanced maternal age and adverse pregnancy outcome: evidence from a large contemporary cohort", in PLoS One.;8(2):e56583.

Krieger JW, and al, Feb 2006, "Effects of variation in protein and carbohydrate intake on body mass and composition during energy restriction: a meta-regression 1", in The American Journal of Clinical Nutrition, 83(2):260-74.

Kristin L. Campbell and Al, (Feb 2012), "Reduced-Calorie Dietary Weight Loss, Exercise, and Sex Hormones in Postmenopausal Women" Randomized Controlled Trial", American Society of Clinical Oncology

Fonken L K., and al, Jun 2013, "Dark nights reverse metabolic disruption caused by dim light at night" in Obesity (Silver Spring), 21(6):1159-64.

Fonken L K., and al, Aug. 2013, "Dim Light at Night Disrupts Molecular Circadian Rhythms and Increases Body Weight Journal of Biological Rhythm, vol. 28 no. 4 262-271

Fuhrman J, Eat to Live: The Revolutionary Formula for Fast and Sustained Weight Little, Brown and Company, NY, Boston, 2003.

Fujioka K, Oct. 2004, "Follow-up of Nutritional and Metabolic Problems After Bariatric Surgery", in Diabetes Care, http://care.diabetesjournals.org.

Hursting SD, and al, 2003, "Calorie restriction, aging, and cancer prevention: mechanisms of action and applicability to humans", in Annual Review of Medicine, 54:131-52.

Largeman FR and Kunes E. ,The Carb Lovers Diet, Time Home Entertainment Inc., NY, 2010.

Layman DK and al, Feb 2003, "A reduced ratio of dietary carbohydrate to protein improves body composition and blood lipid profiles during weight loss in adult women", in The Journal of Nutrition, 133(2):411-7.

Li W., may 2011, "Antioxidants Against Cancer", in http://www.doctoroz.com/videos/antioxidants-against-cancer.

Loyd RA, et al. "Update on the evaluation and management of functional dyspepsia" in American Family Physician, 2011; 83:547

Lowe MR, and Butryn ML, Jul 2007, "Hedonic hunger: a new dimension of appetite?", in Physiology and Behavior, 24;91(4):432-9. .

Lu J, and al, May 2010, "Purple sweet potato color alleviates D-galactose-induced brain aging in old mice by promoting survival of neurons via PI3K pathway and inhibiting cytochrome C-mediated apoptosis", in Brain Pathology, 20(3):598-612.

Lucock M, and Yates Z, Nov 2009, "Folic acid fortification: a double-edged sword", in Current Opinion in Clinical Nutrition and Metabolic Care, 12(6):555-64.

Lundin KE, and Alaedini A., Oct 2012, "Non-celiac gluten sensitivity", in Gastrointestinal endoscopy clinics of north America, 22(4):723-34.

Manson JE, and al, Sep. 1995, "Body weight and mortality among women", in The New-England Journal of Medicine, 14;333(11):677-85.

Marcus et al., 2008, "Comparison of Combined Aerobic and High-Force Eccentric Resistance Exercise With Aerobic Exercise Only for People With Type 2 Diabetes Mellitus. Physical Therapy, 2008; DOI: 10.2522/ptj.20080124.

Martens MK, and al, Dec. 2005, "Why do adolescents eat what they eat? Personal and social environmental predictors of fruit, snack and breakfast consumption among 12-14-year-old Dutch students", in Public Health Nutrition, 8(8):1258-65..

Martin K, and al., Jun 2004, "Estimation of resting energy expenditure considering effects of race and diabetes status", in Diabetes Care, 27(6):1405-11.

Mattes RD, and Dreher ML., 2010, "Nuts and healthy body weight maintenance mechanisms", in Asia Pacific Journal of clinical nutrition, 19(1):137-41.

Maurer-Spurej E., Pittendreigh, Ch., and Misri Sh, Jan 2007, "Platelet serotonin levels support depression scores for women with postpartum depression", in Journal of Psychiatry and Neuroscience, 31 (1): 23-29.

May, L A and al, May 2012, "Prevalence of Cardiovascular Disease Risk Factors among US Adolescents, 1999–2008", in Pediatrics, doi: 10.1542/peds.2011-1082.

McKeith G., Living Food for Health: 12 Natural Superfoods to Transform Your Health, Basic Health Publications Inc., London, 2005.

McGuire, M.T., et al. (1999). "What predicts weight regain in a group of successful weight losers?" In Journal of Consulting and Clinical Psychology, 67 (2), 177–85.

Mclean N., Sep. 2003 " Family involvement in weight control, weight maintenance and weight-loss interventions: a systematic review of randomised trials", in International Journal of Obesity and related metabolic disorders, 27(9):987-1005.

Mei Z, and al, 2012, "Validity of body mass index compared with other body-composition screening indexes for the assessment of body fatness in children and adolescents", in American Journal of Clinical Nutrition;7597–985.

Meule A. and Vögele C., April 2013, "The Psychology of Eating", in Frontiers in Psychology, 4: 215.

Mi Shi and Xiangzhong Zheng, Oct. 2012, "Interactions between the circadian clock and metabolism: there are good times and bad times" in Journal of Molecular call Biology, 45 (1): 61-69.

Mitchell S, Sep 10th 2009, "How Friendship Affects Children's Eating Habits", in Opra.com.1-4.

Mokdad AH, and al, Mar. 2004, " Actual causes of death in the United States, 2000", in JAMA, the Journal of the American Medical Association, 10;291(10):1238-45.

Motl RW, O'Connor PJ, Dishman RK., Aug 2003, "Effect of caffeine on perceptions of leg muscle pain during moderate intensity cycling exercise", in The Journal of Pain, 4(6):316-21.

Mukamal KJ, and al, Jan 2006, "Alcohol consumption and risk of coronary heart disease in older adults: the Cardiovascular Health Study", in Journal of the American Geriatric Society, 54(1):30-7.

Nawrot P, and al, Jan 2003, "Effects of caffeine on human health", in Food Additives and Contaminants, 20(1):1-30

Must A and Anderson SE., 2003, "Effects of obesity on morbidity in children and adolescents", in Nutrition in Clinical Care;6(1):4–12.

Nedeltcheva AV, and al, Oct 2010, "Insufficient sleep undermines dietary efforts to reduce adiposity", in Annals of Internal Medicine, 5;153(7):435-41.

Niemeier HM, and al, Dec 2006, "Fast food consumption and breakfast skipping: predictors of weight gain from adolescence to adulthood in a nationally representative sample", in The Journal of Adolescent health, 39(6):842-9.

Neuhouser ML and al, Jan 1999, "Use of food nutrition labels is associated with lower fat intake", in Journal of the American Dietetic Association, 99(1):45-53.

Noakes M, and al, Jun 2005, "Effect of an energy-restricted, high-protein, low-fat diet relative to a conventional high-carbohydrate, low-fat diet on weight loss, body composition, nutritional status, and markers of cardiovascular health in obese women", in The American Journal of Clinical Nutrition, 81(6):1298-306.

Nogal, P; Lewiński, A, Mar 2008,. "Anorexia Nervosa". In Endokrynologia Polska/Polish Journal of Endocrinology 59 (2): 148–155.

Nordin BE., Jul-Aug 1997, Calcium and osteoporosis, in Nutrition, 13(7-8):664-86.

Obayashi Kand al, Jan 2013, "Exposure to light at night, nocturnal urinary melatonin excretion, and obesity/dyslipidemia in the elderly: a cross-sectional analysis of the HEIJO-KYO study", in The Journal of clinical Endocrinology and Metabolism, 98(1):337-44

Ogden Jane, (March 2009), Understanding the role of life events in weight loss and weight gain, Psychology, Health & Medicine, Vol. 14, No. 2, 239–249.

O'Neill Hill L., (Jan 2013), "Thin is in, but fat might be better", Special to CNN.com

Osganian SK, and al.,Jul-Aug 1996, "Changes in the nutrient content of school lunches: results from the CATCH Eat Smart Food service Intervention", in Preventive Medicine, 25(4):400-12. .

Oz M, "Oz's Two-Day Wonder Cleanse", in http://www.oprah.com/health/Dr-Oz-on-Cleansing-Do-You-Need-a-Cleanse.

Oz M, "Just For Kids", in http://www.oprah.com/health/Just-For-Kids-Daphne-Oz-Dr-Ozs-daughter/1.

Ozdemir1 B. and Al, (January 2013), "How safe is the use of herbal weight-loss products sold over the Internet?" Hum Exp Toxicol vol. 32 no. 1 101-106.

Paavo A., There is a cure for Arthritis, Prentice Hall Press 1988.

Peeake P, Fit to live, Rodale Inc. NY, 2007.

Planck N., 2006, Real Food: What to Eat and Why, Bloomsbury Publishing PLC.

Pollan M., 2008, In Defence Of Food: The Myth Of Nutrition And The Pleasures Of Eating, Penguin Press HC.

Pollan M., 2009, Food Rules: An Eater's Manual, Penguin Books.

Paniagua JA, and al, Jul 2007, "Monounsaturated fat-rich diet prevents central body fat distribution and decreases postprandial adiponectin expression induced by a carbohydrate-rich diet in insulin-resistant subjects", in Diabetes Care.;30(7):1717-23..

Pope L, and Wolf RL., Mar-Apr 2012, "The influence of labeling the vegetable content of snack food on children's taste preferences: a pilot study", in Journal of Nutrition Education and Behavior, 44(2):178-82.

Quintana DS, and al, Aug 2013, "Moderate alcohol intake is related to increased heart rate variability in young adults: Implications for health and well-being", in Psychophysiology. doi: 10.1111/psyp.12134. [Epub ahead of print]

Reilly JJ ,Dorosty AR., 1999, "Epidemic of obesity in UK children" .Lancet 1874, 5-354/

Reilly JJ ,Dorosty AR, Emmett PM., 1999, "Prevalence of overweight and obesity In British children: cohort study", .BMJ.319:1039;

Reinecke A, and al, Jun 2013, "Changes in automatic threat processing precede and predict clinical changes with exposure-based cognitive-behavior therapy for panic disorder", in Biological Psychiatry, 1;73(11):1064-70.

Reinehr T, and Andler W., Oct 2002, "Thyroid hormones before and after weight loss in obesity", in Archives of Disease in Childhood, 87(4):320-3.

Renwick AG.jan 1994, "Intense sweeteners, food intake, and the weight of a body of evidence", in Physiology and Behavior, 55(1):139-43.

Ruesten Von A. and al, 2012; "Association of Sleep Duration with Chronic Diseases in the European Prospective Investigation into Cancer and Nutrition (EPIC)-Potsdam Study" in PloS ONE, 7(1): e30972.

Richards J., and. Gumz L M., June 2013, "Mechanism of the circadian clock in physiology", in American Journal of Physiology Vol. 304no. R1053-R1064.

Rimm EB, and al, Mar 1996, "Review of moderate alcohol consumption and reduced risk of coronary heart disease: is the effect due to beer, wine, or spirits", BMJ. 23;312(7033):731-6.

Ronald J. and al, Sep. 2012, "Trends in Physical Activity, Sedentary Behavior, Diet, and BMI Among US Adolescents, 2001-2009", in Pediatrics, 132:4 606-614

Rosen JC, Reiter J, Orosan P., 1995, "Assessment of body image in eating disorders with the body dysmorphic disorder examination", in Behaviour Research and Therapy 33 (1): 77–84.

Rudolf MCJ ,Sahota P, Barth JH ,et l..(2001) "Increasing prevalence of obesity in primary school children: cohort study", .BMJ,.5–322:1094

Ryan M., 2007, Sports Nutrition for Endurance Athletes, Velo Press.

Sakurai M, and al, Apr 2013, "Sugar-sweetened beverage and diet soda consumption and the 7-year risk for type 2 diabetes mellitus in middle-aged Japanese men", in European Journal of Nutrition, [Epub ahead of print]

Salvy SJ and al, Jan 2011, "Influence of parents and friends on children's and adolescents' food intake and food selection", in The American Journal of Clinical Nutrition, 93(1):87-92.

Sanders RD, and al, Jul 2013, "Perioperative statin therapy for improving outcomes during and after noncardiac vascular surgery", in The Cochrane database of systematic reviews, 3;7:CD009971.

Sawka MN, Cheuvront SN, Carter R 3rd. Jun 2005, "Human water needs", in Nutrition Reviews, 63(6 Pt 2):S30-9.

Schernhammer ES, and al, Dec 2012, "Consumption of artificial sweetener- and sugar-containing soda and risk of lymphoma and leukemia in men and women", in The American Journal of Clinical Nutrition, 96(6):1419-28.

Sherman H., and al, May 2012, "Timed high-fat diet resets circadian metabolism and prevents obesity", in The FASEB Journal, 26(8):3493-502

Sinclair S. Feb 2000, "Male infertility: nutritional and environmental considerations", in Alternative Medicine Review, 5(1):28-38.

Simopoulos AP., Dec 2002, "Omega-3 fatty acids in inflammation and autoimmune diseases", in Journal of the American College of Nutrition, 21(6):495-505.

Skov AR, and al,, May, 1999, "Randomized trial on protein vs. carbohydrate in ad libitum fat reduced diet for the treatment of obesity", in International Journal of Obesity and Related Metabolic Disorders, 23(5):528-36..

Slattery ML and al,July 1998, " Eating patterns and risk of colon cancer" in American Journal of Epidemiology, 1;148(1):4-16.

Smith A., Sep 2002, "Effects of caffeine on human behavior", in Food and Chemical Toxicology, 40(9):1243-55.

Smith AD, and al, Mar 2008, "Is folic acid good for everyone?", in The American Journal of Clinical Nutrition, 87(3):517-33.

Steinberg FM, Bearden MM, Keen CL., Feb 2003, "Cocoa and chocolate flavonoids: implications for cardiovascular health", in Journal of the American Dietetic Association, 103(2):215-23.

Steffens S, Mach F., Nov 2004, "Anti-inflammatory properties of statins", in Seminar in vascular medicine, 4(4):417-22.

Stott DJ, and al, Dec 2008, "Does low to moderate alcohol intake protect against cognitive decline in older people?", in Journal of the American Geriatric Society, 56(12):2217-24.

Strauss R. Jan 2000, "Childhood obesity and self-esteem", in Pediatrics ;105:e15.

Stroebele N and De Castro JM, Sep 2004, "Effect of ambience on food intake and food choice", in Nutrition, 20(9):821-38.

S. N. Blair and J. N. Morris, 2009,"Healthy hearts-and the universal benefits of being physically active: physical activity and health," in Annals of Epidemiology, vol. 19, no. 4, pp. 253–256.

Stunkard AJ and al, Jul 1955, "The night-eating syndrome; a pattern of food intake among certain obese patients", in The American Journal of Medicine, 19(1):78-86.

Sturm R, Oct. 2003, "Increases in clinically severe obesity in the United States, 1986-2000", in Archives of Internal Medicine, 13;163(18):2146-8.

Surén P, and al, Feb 2013, "Association between maternal use of folic acid supplements and risk of autism spectrum disorders in children", in The Journal of the American Medical Association, 13;309(6):570-7.

Svetkey LP, and al, Jan 2005, "Effect of lifestyle modifications on blood pressure by race, sex, hypertension status, and age", in Journal of Human Hypertension, 19(1):21-31.

Sweetman C, and al, Feb 2011, "Characteristics of family mealtimes affecting children's vegetable consumption and liking", in Journal of the American Dietetic Association, 111(2):269-73..

Taheri Sh. and al, 2004, "Short sleep duration is associated with reduced leptin, elevated ghrelin, and increased body mass index" in PLoS Med;1:e62.

Tak NI, and al, Dec. 2010, "The effects of a fruit and vegetable promotion intervention on unhealthy snacks during mid-morning school breaks: results of the Dutch Schoolgruiten Project", in Journal of Human Nutrition and Dietetics, 23(6):609-15.

Teachman BA, and al, Dec. 2008, "Automatic associations and panic disorder: trajectories of change over the course of treatment", in Journal of Consulting and clinical Psychology, 76(6):988-1002.

Temple JL, and al, 2008 May, "Overweight children find food more reinforcing and consume more energy than do nonoverweight children", In The American Journal of Clinical Nutrition, 87(5):1121-7.

Tremblay A, and Chaput JP., Aug 2009, "Adaptive reduction in thermogenesis and resistance to lose fat in obese men", in The British Journal of Nutrition, 102(4):488-92.

Treyzon L. and al, Aug 2008, "A controlled trial of protein enrichment of meal replacements for weight reduction with retention of lean body mass" , in Nutrition Journal, 7:23 Published online 10.1186/1475-2891-7-23.

Trzesniewski KH and al, Mar 2006, "Low self-esteem during adolescence predicts poor health, criminal behavior, and limited economic prospects during adulthood", in Development Psychology, 42(2):381-90.

Tschiesche J, Not Just Sandwiches: *5 Ways To Improve Your Child's Lunchbox*, Random House, London, 2012.

Tucker KL, and al, Oct 2006, "Colas, but not other carbonated beverages, are associated with low bone mineral density in older women: The Framingham Osteoporosis Study", in The American Journal of clinical Nutrition, 84(4):936-42.

Tylk T, march 2011 "Women's Body Image Based More On Others' Opinions Than Their Own Weight" in Medical News Today, http://www.medicalnewstoday.com/releases/220591.php.

Umpierre D. and al, May 2011, " Physical activity advice only or structured exercise training and association with HbA1c levels in type 2 diabetes: a systematic review and meta-analysis", in JAMA, the Journal of the American Medical Association, 4;305(17):1790-9.

Vanhees K, and al., Jul. 2013, "You are what you eat, and so are your children: the impact of micronutrients on the epigenetic programming of offspring", in Cellular and Molecular Life Sciences, [Epub ahead of print].

Vastag B, Mar 2004, "Obesity Is Now on Everyone's Plate", in JAMA, the journal of the American Medical Association, 10;291(10):1186-8.

Vincent A, and Fitzpatrick LA., Nov 2000, "Soy isoflavones: are they useful in menopause?", in Mayo Clinic Proceedings, 75(11):1174-84.

Volkert D, and al, May 1991, "[Malnutrition in old age--results of the Bethany nutrition study]", [Article in German], in Therapeutische Umschau, 48(5):312-5.

Volta U, and al, Sep 2013, " Non-celiac gluten sensitivity: questions still to be answered despite increasing awareness", in Cellular and Molecular Immunology, 10(5):383-9.

Vorona RD, and al, Jan 2005, "Overweight and obese patients in a primary care population report less sleep than patients with a normal body mass index", in Achieves of Internal Medicine, 10;165(1):25-30.

Zafra C. and al, (august 2010), "Testing a new cognitive behavioural treatment for obesity: A randomized controlled trial with three-year follow-up", in Behav Res Ther. 48(8): 706–713.

Zinczenko D, Goulding M, 2010, Eat This, Not That! Thousands of Simple Food Swaps that Can Save You 10, 20, 30 Pounds--or More! Rodale Inc.

Gary L.Wenk, Ph.D., author of Your Brain on Food (Oxford, 2010); http://faculty.psy.ohio-state.edu/wenk/

Wardle J, and al, Apr 2004"Increasing children's acceptance of vegetables; a randomized trial of parent-led exposure", in Appetite, 40(2):155-62.

Westerterp-Plantenga MS, and al, Jul 2005, "Body weight loss and weight maintenance in relation to habitual caffeine intake and green tea supplementation", in Obesity Research, 13(7):1195-204.

Williams DP, and al, Mar. 1992, "Body fatness and risk for elevated blood pressure, total cholesterol, and serum lipoprotein ratios in children and adolescents", in American Journal of Public Health, 82(3):358-63.

Wilson SM, Sato AF. (July 1 2013), "Stress and Paediatric Obesity: What We Know and Where To Go" in Stress Health, David Zinczenko (Author) › Visit Amazon's David Zinczenko Page.

Wing, R. R. and Phelan, S. 2005, "Long-term weight loss maintenance", in American Journal of Clinical Nutrition, 82 (suppl), 222S-225S.

Witte AV, and al, Jun 2013, "Long-Chain Omega-3 Fatty Acids Improve Brain Function and Structure in Older Adults", Cerebral Cortex, [Epub ahead of print].

Whitaker RC, and al, 1997, "Predicting obesity in young adulthood from childhood and parental obesity" in New England Journal of Medicine;37(13):869–873.

Wroten KC, and al, Oct. 2012," Resemblance of dietary intakes of snacks, sweets, fruit, and vegetables among mother-child dyads from low income families", in Appetite, 59(2):316-23.

(World Health Organization, Obesity, preventing and managing the global epidemic, Report of the WHO consultation of obesity. Geneva: World Health Organization, 1997).

National Adult office, Tackling obesity in England. Report by the Comptroller and Auditor General London: The Stationary Office, 2001.

Dietary Reference Intakes for Water, Potassium, Sodium, Chloride, and Sulfate, Panel on Dietary Reference Intakes for Electrolytes and Water, Standing Committee on the Scientific Evaluation of Dietary Reference Intakes ISBN: 0-309-53049-0, 640 pages, 6 x 9, National Academy of Sciences, 2004.

Indigestion. National Institute for Diabetes and Digestive and Kidney Diseases. http://digestive.niddk.nih.gov/ddiseases/pubs/indigestion/index.aspx. Accessed Oct. 17, 2011.

World Health Organization, http://www.who.int/topics/en/

AMA American Medical Association, http://www.ama-assn.org/ama/home.page

Policy and action for cancer prevention — food, nutrition, and physical activity: a global perspective. Washington (DC): World Cancer Research Fund/American Institute for Cancer Research; 2009. p. 86. Available: www.dietandcancerreport.org

Supplement to "F as in fat: how obesity policies are failing America, 2009" obesity-related legislation action in States, update. Washington (DC): Trust for America's Health. Available: http://healthyamericans.org/reports/obesity2009/StateSupplement2009.pdf.

Mind

Abu Shakra M. and al, (1999). "Quality of life in systemic lupus erythematosus: a controlled study'" in Journal of Rheumatology, 26, 306-309.

Abu-Shakra, M. (2008). "Do improved survival rates of patients with systemic lupus erythematosus reflect a global trend?" in Journal of Rheumatology, 35, 1906-1908

After, A., Hatav, Y., Weizman, A., and Tiano, 1998, S. Psychiatry of the Child and Adolescent: Body Image, Dionon Press, Tel Aviv University. (In Hebrew).

Ahsian N, The Crystal Ally Cards,S Heaven & Earth Publishing, Marshfield, 1995.

Amossy R. 1999, Image se soi dans ke discours. La construction de l'ethos, Geneve, Delachaux et Niestle. (In French).

Anderson JW and al, Mar. 2008, "Blood pressure response to transcendental meditation: a meta-analysis", in American Journal of Hypertension, 21(3):310-6.

Andrea C and Andrea S, Heart of the Mind: Engaging Your Inner Power to change with NLP, Real People Press, Utah, 1989.

Andreas C and Andreas S., Change your Mind – and keep the change, Advanced NLP submodalities inerventions, Real People Press, Utah, 1987.

Andreas S. and Faulkner Ch., The NLP Comprehensive Training Team NLP the new Technology of achievement, William Morrow and Company INC, New York, 1994.

Andreas S. and Faulkner Ch., ed. NLP, The New Technology of Achievement, William Morrow and Company, INC, NY, 1994.

Arias AJ., and al, 2006, "Systematic review of the efficacy of meditation techniques as treatments for medical illness", in Journal of Alternative Complementary Medicine, 12(8):817-32.

University of Maryland Medical Center
Follow us: @UMMC on Twitter | MedCenter on Facebook.

Aristote, 1989, Rethorique des passions, postface de Michel Meyer, Paris, Rivages. (In French).

Aristotle, The Physics, Books I-IV, Loeb Classical Library, No. 228, 1957.

Ashby F, Gregory and John M, Ennis "The role of the Basal Ganglia in Category Learning", in Psychology of Learning and Motivation 46 (2006), 1-36.

Ashby F, Gregory, Turner O and J C Horvits, "Cortical and basal Ganglia Contributions to Habit Learning and Automaticity" John M, Ennis Trends in Cognitive Sciences 14 (2010), 15-208.

Austin J L. , How to Do Things with Words, Oxford, NY, 1962.

Baird, Forrest E.; Walter Kaufmann, 2008, From Plato to Derrida. Upper Saddle River, New Jersey: Pearson Prentice Hal.

Bamberger, Bernard J. Fallen angels : soldiers of Satan's realm (1. paperback ed. ed.). Philadelphia, Pa.: Jewish Publ. Soc. of America, 2006.

Bandler R,, Grinder J , The Structure of Magic I: A Book about Language and Therapy, Science and Behavior Book, 1975.

Bandler R and Grinder J, Frogs into Princes, Real People Press, Utah, 1979.

Bandler R, Using your Brain – for a Change, Real People Press, Utah, 1985.

Bandler R and Grinder J., Patterns of the Hypnotic techniques of Milton H. Erickson, M.D. Meta Publications Inc, Cupertino, CA.

Başar E, and al, 2013, "Brain's alpha, beta, gamma, delta, and theta oscillations in neuropsychiatric diseases: proposal for biomarker strategies", in Supplements to Clinical

Neurophysiology, 62:19-54.

Bateson G, Step to an Ecology of Mind Collected Essays in Anthropology, Psychiatry, Evolution, and Epistemology. University Of Chicago Press, 1972

Benor DJ, and al, Nov-Dec 2009, "Pilot study of emotional freedom techniques, wholistic hybrid derived from eye movement desensitization and reprocessing and emotional freedom technique, and cognitive behavioral therapy for treatment of test anxiety in university students", in Explore (NY), 5(6):338-40.

Benson H and Klipper M. Z and, The Relaxation Response, Publishers Inc., NY, 1975.

Becker T, Jan 2012, "Hormesis and the limbic brain", in www.gettingstronger.org.

Ben-Israel N, "Vianna's ThetaHealingTM Practitioner Manuel", 2012, in Hebrew.

Bernatsky S, Boivin JF, and al., 2010, "Mortality in systemic lupus erythematosus" in Arthritis Rheum.;54:2550–2557. doi: 10.1002/art.21955.

Banmen J, March 2002, "The Satir Model: Yesterday and Today", in Contemporary Family Theory, 24 (1).

Blanchette Ph., 1995, La Pragmatique d'Austine a Goffman, Paris, Bertrand-Lacoste. (In French).

Bodenhamer B and Hall M, Adventures with Time Lines", Meta Publications, Capitola, California, 1998.

Bolocofsky DN, Spinler D, Coulthard-Morris L., Jan 1985, "Effectiveness of hypnosis as an adjunct to behavioral weight management", in Journal of Clinical Psychology. 41(1):35-41.

Bonnet Ch., and Tamine J., Juin 1982, "La comprehension des metaphors chez les enfants, une hypothese et quelques implicayions pedagogiques", L'Information Grammaticale, 14, Paris, 17-23. (In French).

Booth C Wayne, 1970, "Distance et point de vue, Essai de classification", in Poetique, 4, 511-524. (In French).

Borg GA., 1982, "Psychophysical bases of perceived exertion", in Medicine and Science in Sports and Exercise, 14(5):377-81.

Bosanac S, Latin D, Mikolić P, Discourse Analysis: Spoken Language, Department of English Faculty of Philosophy University of Zagreb, Zagreb, 2009.

Bouras, N.; Holt, G. Psychiatric and Behavioral Disorders in Intellectual and Developmental Disabilities (2nd ed.). Cambridge University Press, 2007.

Brennen B Hands of Light: A Guide to Healing Through the Human Energy Field, Bantam books, NY, 1988.

Brown RP and Gerbarg PL., Aug. 2009, " Yoga breathing, meditation, and longevity", in Annals of the New York Academy of Sciences, 1172:54-62.

Butto N, Medicina universale e il settimo senso, Edizioni Mediterranee, 2004. (In Italian).

Byrne R, The Secret, TS Production, Luxembourg, 2006.

Byron L., Pucelik F., Magic NLP Demystified, a pragmatic guide to Communication and Change, Metamorphous Press, Portland, Oregon, 1982.

Byron K, Living what is, Three Rivers Press, NY, 2002.

Cahn BR., and Polich J. Mar 2006, "Meditation states and traits: EEG, ERP, and neuroimaging studies", in Psychological Bulletin, 132(2):180-211.

Callahan, R. Five minute phobia cure. Wilmington, DE: Enterprise Publishing, 1985.

Callahan, R. J., & Callahan, J.. 1996,. Thought Field Therapy (TFT) and trauma: Treatment and theory. Indian Wells, CA: Thought Field Therapy Training Center.

Callahan R. Tapping the Healer Within: Using Thought Field Therapy to Instantly Conquer Your Fears, Anxieties, and Emotional Distress. New York, NY, USA: McGraw-Hill; 2000.

Cameron-Bandler L, The Emotional Hostage: Rescuing Your Emotional Life, Real People Press, 1986.

Carmody TP, and al, May 2008, "Hypnosis for smoking cessation: a randomized trial", in Nicotine and Tobacco Research, 10(5):811-8.

Chew M., and van der Weyden, M.B. (2003). "Chronic illness: the burden and the dream" in Medical Journal of Australia, 179, 229-30.

Chopra D, Oct. 2009, "5 Rules for timeless living", in Oprah.com

Church, D., Brooks, A. J. 2010, "The effect of a brief EFT (Emotional Freedom Techniques) self-intervention on anxiety, depression, pain and cravings in healthcare workers, in Integrative Medicine: A Clinician's Journal, 9(5), 40-44.

Church D, Yount G, Brooks AJ., Oct 2012, "The effect of emotional freedom techniques on stress biochemistry: a randomized controlled trial", in The Journal of Nervous and Mental Disease, 200(10):891-6.

Clark, P. J., and al, Apr 2011, "Genetic influences on exercise-induced adult hippocampal neurogenesis across 12 divergent mouse strains", in Genes, Brain and Behavior, 10: 345–353.

Colzanto, L S; van Wouwe, N C; Lavender, T J; & Hommel, B (2006). "Intelligence and cognitive flexibility: Fluid intelligence correlates with feature "unbinding" across perception and action.". Psychonomic Bulletin & Review 13: 1043–1048. doi:10.3758/BF0321392

Colzato, L S; van Leeuwen, P; van den Wildenberg, W; Hommel, B (2010). "DOOM'd to switch: superior cognitive flexibility in players of first person shooter games". Front. Psychology. doi:10.3389/fpsyg.2010.00008.

Craig G. The EFT Manual, Energy. Santa Rosa, California, USA: Psychology Press; 2008.

Craig G., "The proper way to use EFT for hurt feelings", in www.emofree.com.

Das L, S, Eight steps to enlightenment: Awakening the Buddha within: Tibetan Buddhism for the Western World, Broadway Books, NY, 1997.

Davison, Gerald C. . Abnormal Psychology. Toronto: Veronica Visentin, 2008.

Derrida J, 1978, "points out Foucault's debt to Artaud in his essay "La parole soufflée," in Derrida, Writing and Difference, trans. Alan Bass p. 326n.26.

Descartes R, Cottingham J editor, Descartes: Meditations on First Philosophy: With Selections from the Objections and Replies, Cambridge University Press, UK, 1996.

Dias E., "The power of habit", in http://personaltraining.showmethefitness.com/articles_by_eduardo/power_of_habits.html, 2009.

Dilts, R., Grinder, J., Delozier, J., and Bandler, R. Neuro-Linguistic Programming: Volume I: The Study of the Structure of Subjective Experience., Cupertino, CA: Meta Publications. 1980.

Dilts R.B., visionary Leadership Skills, Creating a World which people Want to belong, Meta Publications, Capitols, California 1996

Dilts R.B, Halbom T, Smith S., Beliefs Pathways to Health & Well-being, Metamorphous Press, Portland, 1990.

Dilts R.B, NLP University, Santa Cruz, CA, 2011, in www.NLPU.com

Ducrot O.1984, Le dire et le dit, Paris, Minuit. (In French).

Duhigg Ch., The Power of Habit, Random House Inc., NY, 2012.

Dusek JA and Benson H, Mar. 2009, " Mind-body medicine: a model of the comparative clinical impact of the acute stress and relaxation responses", in Minnesota Medicine, ;92(5):47-50..

Dworkin PH., Feb 1988, "The preschool child: developmental themes and clinical issues", in Current Problems in Pediatrics, 18(2):73-134.

Edvardsson JD, Sandman PO, Rasmussen BH., Jul 2003, "Meanings of giving touch in the care of older patients: becoming a valuable person and professional", in Journal of Clinical Nursing, 12(4):601-9.

Eemeren F., H van and al, 1996, Fundementals of Argumentation Theory, A handbook of Historical Backgrounds and Contemporary Develipments, ahwah, New Jersey, Lawrence Erlbaum Associates Publishers.

Epstein M., Dalai Lama XIV (Foreword), 1996, Thoughts Without A Thinker: Psychotherapy From A Buddhist Perspective, Basic Books.

Erickson M., H., 1991, In His Own Voice, edited by Jay Haley and co-edited by Madeleine Richeport, New York, WW Norton & Company.

Faulkner CH, Gerling K., Schmidth G., Halborn T., Smith S., McDonald R., A pocket guide to NLP, the new technology of achievement, Nightgale-conant Corporation, Illinois, 1991.

Feinstein D, Eden D and Graig G, The Promise of Energy Psychology Revolutionary Tools for Dramatic Personal Change, Penguin Group Inc., NY, 2005.

Feinstein, D. 2012, "Acupoint stimulation in treating psychological disorders: Evidence of efficacy", in Review of General Psychology, 16, 364-380

Foster C., al, Jan 2008, "The talk test as a marker of exercise training intensity", in Journal of Cardiopulmonary Rehabilitation, 28(1):24-30.

Foucault M., Archaeology of Knowledge. Routledge, Paris, 1972.

Frackowiak R S J and al, Human brain Function, Academic Press, San Diego, 1997.

Gandhi M., John Dear, 2002, Essential Writings (Modern Spiritual Masters), Orbis Books. (first published June 1970).

Grice P., 1970, "Logique et conversation", in Communication, 30. (In French)

Grinder J., and Bandler, R., The Structure of Magic II (1st ed.). California: Science and Behavior Books, 1976.

Grinder J and Bandler R, Trance-formations, NLP and the structure of Hypnosis, Real People Press, Utah, 1981.

Gardes-Tamine J., 1996, La Rethorique, Paris, Armand Colin. (In French).

Gloor P., and al, Aug 1982, "The role of the limbic system in experiential phenomena of temporal lobe epilepsy", in Annals of Neurology, 12(2):129-44.

Gloor P, The Temporal Lobe and Limbic System, Oxford University Press, USA, 1997.

Golan M, " The Power of Theta Brainwave to Heal", in about.com, 2013.

Golombek U., Nov. 2001, " [Progressive muscle relaxation (PMR) according to Jacobson in a department of psychiatry and psychotherapy - empirical results]", in Psychiatrische Praxis,. 28(8):402-4.

Hanh T N, The Miracle of Mindfulness, Beacon, Boston, 1975.

Haley J, Jay Haley on Dr. Milton H. Erickson, Brunner-Rutledge, London, 1993.

Halevi J, The Kuzari: An Argument for the Faith of Israel, Schocken Books Inc. NY, 1964.

Hamburg J and al, 2004, "The Effects of a Laban-Based Movement Program with Music on Measures of Balance and Gait in Older Adults", in Activities, Adaptation & Aging, vol 28, Issue 1, 17-33.

Hariri AR, Bookheimer SY, Mazziotta JC.. Jan 2000, "Modulating emotional responses: effects of a neocortical network on the limbic system", in Neuroreport. 17;11(1):43-8.

Harper, D,. "communication". Online Etymology Dictionary. Retrieved 2013-06-23.

Herrick J. A. 2007, Argumentation: Understanding and Shaping Arguments, Strata Publishing. (First published November 1st 1994).

Hertenstein MJ, and al, Aug 2006, "Touch communicates distinct emotions", in Emotion, 6(3):528-33.

Hertenstein MJ, Keltner D. Jan 2011, "Gender and the Communication of Emotion Via Touch", in Sex Roles, 64(1-2):70-80.

Hodgson J., Mastering Movement: The Life and Work of Rudolf Laban, Routledge, NY, 2001.

Inman M, May 2011, "A Rosetta Stone for Brain Waves", in PloS Biology, 9(5) e1001063.

Jain S., and al, Feb. 2007, "A randomized controlled trial of mindfulness meditation versus relaxation training: effects on distress, positive states of mind, rumination, and distraction", in Annals of Behavioral Medicine, 33(1):11-21.

James W, The Principles of Psychology, Vol. 1 Dover Publications, NY, 1950.

Jordan MM and al, Aug 2013, " Thinking through every step: how people with spinal cord injuries relearn to walk", in Qualitative Health Research;23(8):1027-41. doi: 10.1177/1049732313494119.

Joseph R., Limbic System: Amygdala, Hippocampus, Hypothalamus, Septal Nuclei, Cingulate, Emotion, Memory, Sexuality, Language, Dreams, Hallucinations, Unconscious Mind, University Press, 2011.

Jourard, S. M. Self-disclosure: An experimental analysis of the transparent self. New York: Wiley-Interscience, 1971.

Karatzias T, and al, Jun 2011, "A controlled comparison of the effectiveness and efficiency of two psychological therapies for posttraumatic stress disorder: eye movement desensitization and reprocessing vs. emotional freedom techniques", in Journal of Nervous and mental Disease, 199(6):372-8.

Kerbrat-Orecchioni C.,1986, L'Implicite, Paris, Armand Colin. (In French).

Kirsch I, Montgomery G, Sapirstein G.. Apr 1995, "Hypnosis as an adjunct to cognitive-behavioral psychotherapy: a meta-analysis", in Journal of Consulting and clinical Psychology, 63(2):214-20.

Konefal J, Duncan RC, Reese MA., Jun 1992, "Neurolinguistic programming training, trait anxiety, and locus of control", in Psychological Reports, 70(3 Pt 1):819-32.

Korzybski A, Science and Sanity: An Introduction to Non-Aristotelian Systems and General Semantics, Institute of General Semantics, New Jersey, 1995.

Kraus KS, Canlon B., Jun 2012, "Neuronal connectivity and interactions between the auditory and limbic systems. Effects of noise and tinnitus", in Hearing Research, 288(1-2):34-46.

Lally Ph and al,)ct. 2010, "How are habits formed: Modelling habit formation in the real world", in European Journal of Social Psychology, 40, 6 pp. 998–1009

Larzelere MM; Jones GN, (December 2008), "Stress and Health", in Primary care, Volume 35, Issue 4

LeDoux J., Oct 2003, "The emotional brain, fear, and the amygdala", in Cellular and Molecular Neurobiology, 23(4-5):727-38.

Light KC, Grewen KM, Amico JA., April 2005, "More frequent partner hugs and higher oxytocin levels are linked to lower blood pressure and heart rate in premenopausal women", in Biological Psychology, 69(1):5-21.

MacLean P.D, The Triune Brain in Evolution: Role in Paleocerebral Functions, Springer, 1990.

Mahncke HW, Bronstone A, Merzenich MM., 2006,"Brain plasticity and functional losses in the aged: scientific bases for a novel intervention", in Progress in Brain Research, 157:81-109.

Marcel G, "Being and Having", Marcel Press, 2007.

Nigel J.T. T Ph.D. , Aug. 1998, " The Study of Imagination as an Approach to Consciousness", Paper presented at the Inaugural Conference of the Society for the

Multidisciplinary Study of Consciousness, California State University, Los Angeles., San Francisco.

Nirula A and Nirual R, The joy of Reiki, Full Circle, Delhi, 1997.

Patterson DR, Jensen MP., Jul 2003, "Hypnosis and clinical pain", in Psychological Bulletin, 129(4):495-521.

Perelman Ch., and Olbrechts-Tyteca L., 1992, Traite de L'Argumentation, La nouvell rhetorique, Bruxelles, Edition de l'Unoiversite de Bruxelles. (First edition in 1958). (In French)

Perelman Ch.,1977, L'empire rhetorique: Retorique et Argumentation, Paris, Vrin. (In French).

Peniston EG, Kulkosky PJ., Apr 1989, "Alpha-theta brainwave training and beta-endorphin levels in alcoholics", in Alcoholism, Clinical and experimental research, 13(2):271-9.

Johnson, R. H., 2000, Manifest Rationality: A Pragmatic Theory of Argument.

Langer E J, and Moldoveanu M (2000), "The construct of Mindfulness" in Journal of Social Issues, 56, 1-9.

Markakis, E.A. and Swanson LW, 1997, "Spatiotemporal patterns of secretomotor neuron generation in the parvicellular neuroendocrine system", in Brain Research. Review. , 24:255-291.

Mizes J S and Bonifazi D Z (2001) "Primary preventions of eating disorders: a noble calling or an unrealistic idea?" in Cognitive and behavioral Practice, 8, 246-248.

PESSANHA, José Américo Motta, (1989), "A Teoria da Argumentação ou nova retórica" (The Theory of Argumentation or New Rhethoric) In CARVALHO, Maria Cecília de. (Org.). Paradigmas Filosóficos da Atualidade (Philosophic Paradigms of the Atuality), Campinas: Papirus, pp. 221-247.

Perelman, Ch., 1969. "The Rational and the Reasonable." In Chaim Perelman, The New Rhetoric and the Humanities: Essays on Rhetoric and its Applications. London: Reidel.

Petersen, C., 2002, "More than a mirror: The ethics of therapist self-disclosure", in . Psychotherapy: Theory, Research, Practice, Training, 19(1), 21-31.

Plantin Ch., 1996, L'Argumentation, Paris, Le Seuil. (In French).

Plantin C., Doury M., Traverso V.,2000, Les Emotions dans les interactions, Presse Universitaires de Lyon. (In French).

Plato, 2003, The Republic, Penguin Classics. (first published 1920).

Raz N., Lindenberger U., Rodrigue K., et al Regional brain changes in aging healthy adults: general trends, individual differences and modifiers. Cereb Cortex. 2005;15:1676–1689.

Reinhard J and al, June 2012, "The Effects of Clinical Hypnosis versus Neurolinguistic Programming (NLP) before External Cephalic Version (ECV): A Prospective Off-Centre Randomised, Double-Blind, Controlled Trial", in Evidence- Based Complementary and Alternative Medicine, 626740. doi: 10.1155/2012/626740.

Rimmon-Kenan Sh., Narrative fiction:Contemporary Poetics, Methuen, London and NY, 1983.

Rosen S., My Voice Will Go With You: The Teaching Tales of Milton H. Erickson, WW Norton & Company: New York, 1991.

Sallivan P F (1995) "Mortality in anorexia nervosa" in American Journal of Psychiatry, 152, 1073-1074.

Satir, V. The new peoplemaking. Palo Alto, CA: Science and Behavior Books, 1988.

Satir, V., Banmen, J., Gerber, J., & Gomori, M. The Satir model: Family therapy and beyond. Palo Alto, CA: Science and Behavior Books., 1991.

"Who Virginia Was and Why She Mattered," Virginia Satir Global Network, Retrieved November 26, 2012

Scott, W A (1962). "Cognitive complexity and cognitive flexibility". American Sociological Association 25: 405–414.

Schwarzenegger A., Petre P, Total Recall: My Unbelievably True Life Story, Simon & Schuster, NY, 2012.

Simi, N. L., & Mahalik, J. R. , 1997, "Comparison of feminist versus psychoanalytic/dynamic and other therapists on self-disclosure", in Psychology of Women Quarterly, 21, 465–483.

Slater VE. Sep 1995, "Toward an understanding of energetic healing, Part 1: Energetic structures", in Journal of Holistic Nursing, 13(3):209-24.

Spechler D, Apr 2013, "How an Extra Touch Can Improve Your Health", in The Oprah Magazine.

Stapleton P and al, Jul 2013, "Depression Symptoms Improve after Successful Weight Loss with Emotional Freedom Techniques", in ISRN Psychiatry. 2013; 2013: 573532.

Steinbach AM, Jan 1984, "Neurolinguistic programming: a systematic approach to change", in Canadian Family physician Medicin de famille Canadien, 30:147-50.

Stevenson M., 2004, Learn Hypnosis... Now!, Liquid Mirror Enterprises, 2004.

Stevenson M., 2007, Time Techniques Practitioner Training, Time Integration for Maximum Empowerment, Transform Destiny, CA USA.

Stevenson M., Transform Destiny NLP Practitioner Certification Training Manuel, V1.2, 2007.

Stewart M, T, (November 2004), "Light of Body Image Treatment, Acceptance through Mindfulness", in Behavior Modification, Vol 28 No 6 , Sage Publications.

Stibal V, Theta Healing Diseases and Disorders, Hay House, Idaho, 2008.

Stibal V, Theta Healing: Introducing an Extraordinary Energy Healing Modality, 2010.

Swanson L.W., 1983, "The hippocampus and the concept of the limbic system", In Neurobiology of the Hippocampus, W. Siefert (ed.), Academic Press, New York, pp. 3-19.

Tad James. Wyatt Woodmalls, Time Line Therapy and the Basis of Personality, Meta Publications, California, 1988.

Tolle Eckhart, A new Earth, Awaking to your Life's Purpose, Penguin Group, NY, 2005.

Thomas Nigel J.T., (August 1998), "The Study of Imagination as an Approach to Consciousness", Paper presented at the Inaugural Conference of the Society for the Multidisciplinary Study of Consciousness, San Francisco.

Tanzi R E, Copr D.,, Super Brain: Unleashing the Explosive Power of Your Mind to Maximize Health, Happiness, and Spiritual Well-Being, Harmony Books, NY, 2012.

Tosey, P., Mathison, J., Introducing Neuro-Linguistic Programming Centre for Management Learning & Development, School of Management, University of Surrey, 2006.

Uramoto, K. M., and al, (1999). "Trends in the incidence and mortality of systemic lupus erythematosus 1950-1992" in Arthritis & Rheumatism, 42, 46-50.

Varnado-Sullivan P J and Zucker N, (Nov 2004),"The body logic program for adolescents, A treatment Manual for the Prevention of Eating Disorders", in Behavior Modification, vo28, no 6, 854-875) Sage Publications.

Virtue D, Assertiveness for Earth Angels, Hay House Inc., 2013.

Ward, K., May 2012, "Virginia Satir: Famous Trailblazer for Compassionate Living," Hubpages.com.

Whittaker, S., May 2007, "Secret attraction" in The Montreal Gazette.

Winnicott, D. W., 1965, Maturational Processes and the Facilitating Environment: Studies in the Theory of Emotional Development, London: Hogarth Press.

Weiss B L Many Lives, Many Masters, Simon & Schuster Inc., NY, 1988

Weiss B L, Through Time Into Healing: Discovering the Power of Regression Therapy to Erase Trauma and Transform Mind, Body and Relationships, Simon & Schuster Inc., NY, 1993.

Xiong GL, Doraiswamy PM, Aug 2009, "Does meditation enhance cognition and brain plasticity?", in Annals of the NY academy of Sciences, 1172:63-9.

Yazdany J, and al, (2008) "Validation of the systemic lupus erythematosus activity questionnaire in a large observational cohort" in Arthritis Rheum. 2008;59:136–143. doi: 10.1002/art.23238.

Yelin E, and al (2007) "Work dynamics among persons with systemic lupus erythematous" in. Arthritis Rheum. 2007;57:56–63. doi: 10.1002/art.22481.

Zur O., 2011, "Self-Disclosure & Transparency in Psychotherapy and Counseling: To Disclose or Not to Disclose, This is the Question", Retrieved November/11/2013 from http://www.zurinstitute.com/selfdisclosure1.html

Hypnotherapy Scripts (Havens & Walters), University of Maryland Medical Center, Relaxation techniques, may 2013.

National Center for Complementary and Alternative Medicine (NCCAM) 2013 http://nccam.nih.gov/health/stress/relaxation.htm.

University of Maryland Medical Center (UMMC), http://umm.edu 2011.

Marina Rose, School of DNA Theta Healing ® Los Angeles, http://www.dnathetahealing.com. 2013.

White Light Healing Chakra Meditation – For You and Humanity - See more at: http://www.wellbeingalignment.com, 2013.

Advanced Psychic development - amplify intuitive and healing skills Theta Healing® Rainbow Children/ Adult , Alexandra P. Brown (2013) http://www.thetahealingacademy.com/our-team.html 2013 by Sandra (Musser) Weaver, 2012-spiritual-growth-prophecies.com

http://www.starchildren.info/rainbow.html, 2007-Nikki Pattillo.

"Go Beyond 'The Secret' - Oprah.com" in oprah.com. Retrieved November 8, 2010.

A Course in Miracles: Text, Workbook for Students, Manual for Teachers, Viking Penguin; second edition, 1996.

"External Cephalic Version (Version) for Breech Position", in WebMD, 2013, http://www.webmd.com.

ABOUT THE AUTHOR

Dr. Anat Feldman is a health consultant and a personal trainer. She holds a Ph.D in Nutritional Science from AIU, (Atlantic International University), a Masters in French Culture and Argumentation from Tel-Aviv University, and a B.Ed. in Physical Education from Wingate Institute. For the last 20 years, using the Gymind method she has developed, Dr. Feldman has guided children and adults on their path for a better and healthier life. She currently lives with her husband and three sons in Israel. This is her first book.

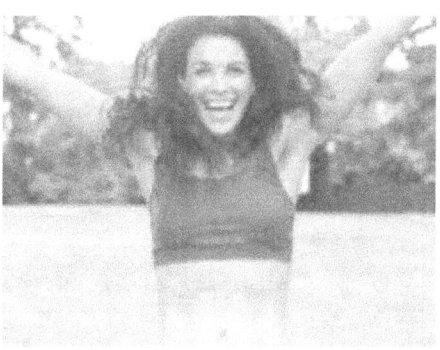